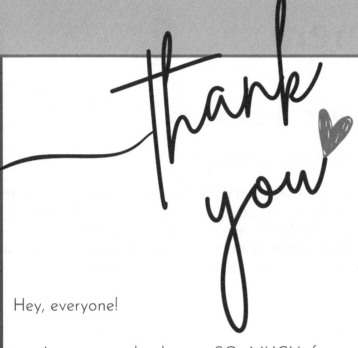

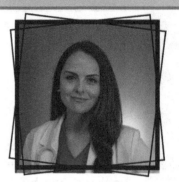

Hey, everyone!

I want to thank you <u>SO MUCH</u> for purchasing my notes on fluid and electrolytes. I hope you find them helpful.

I know this topic can sometimes be overwhelming and frustrating. My goal in creating these notes for you was to try to make your studying process easier. Each chapter includes my review notes, which highlight key concepts to know for exams, fun illustrations, mnemonics, worksheets, and test questions with answers and rationales.

Again, thank you for your purchase and for studying with me. I love you all, and I promise that all of this hard work you are doing will pay off. Never give up on your dreams!

Connect with Me:

- **YouTube**-RegisteredNurseRN
- **Website**-RegisteredNurseRN.com
- **Instagram**-registerednursern_com
- **Facebook**-RegisteredNurseRNs
- **TeeSpring**-RegisteredNurseRN
- **TikTok**-@registerednursern.com
- **Twitter**-NursesRN

So, let's get started...

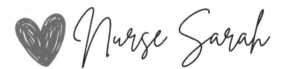

Nurse Sarah

Copyright & Disclaimer

Table of
CONTENTS

1 Fluid Compartments, Movement of Fluids and Solutes, & IV Fluids

2 Fluid Balance: Hormones & Body Systems

Table of CONTENTS

3 Electrolytes

4 Acid-Base Imbalances

Table of
CONTENTS

5 Fluid Volume Disorders

Labs to Know

Metabolic Panel

- **Glucose:** 70–100 mg/dL
- **Calcium:** 8.5–10.5 mg/dL
- **Chloride:** 95-105 mEq/L
- **Magnesium:** 1.5-2.5 mg/dL
- **Phosphorus:** 2.5–4.5 mg/dL
- **Potassium:** 3.5-5 mEq/L
- **Sodium:** 135-145 mEq/L
- **BUN:** 5-20 mg/dL
- **Serum creatinine:** 0.6–1.2 mg/dL
- **Total Protein:** 6.2–8.2 g/dL
- **Albumin:** 3.4–5.4 g/dL
- **Bilirubin:** 0.1-1 mg/dL (less 1)
- **ALP:** 40-120 U/L
- **ALT:** 7 to 56 U/L
- **AST:** 10-40 U/L

This blood test can be ordered as a **BMP (basic metabolic panel)** or CMP **(comprehensive metabolic panel).** CMP will check everything a BMP does, but it also includes liver function tests (noted in red).

Complete Blood Count

- **WBC:** 5,000–10,000 per mcL
  - CBC with differential: assesses **5 types of WBCs:**
    - **Monocytes:** (4-13%)
    - **Eosinophils:** (1-5%)
    - **Neutrophils:** (40-70%)
    - **Basophils:** (0.1-2%)
    - **Lymphocytes:** (20-40%)
- **RBC:** 4.5–5.5 million cells/mcL
  - RBC indices: further looks at RBC (size, amount of hemoglobin etc.)
    - **MCV:** 80-100 fl
    - **MCH:** 27-33 pg per cell
    - **MCHC:** 33-36 g/dL
    - **RDW:** 11-15%
- **Platelets:** 150,000–400,000 per mcL
  - **MPV:** platelet volume 7-10 fl
- **Hemoglobin:**
  - 12–16 g/dL **(female)**
  - 14–18 g/dL **(male)**
- **Hematocrit:**
  - 37 – 47% **(female)**
  - 42 – 52% **(male)**

If results on the CBC are abnormal, a peripheral smear may be ordered. This will look at the morphology (this means the form or the shape of the cell).

Coagulation

- **PT (prothrombin time):** 10-12 seconds
- **INR (international normalized ratio):** < 1
  - When a patient is taking the anticoagulant Warfarin, the INR should be **2-3.**
  - The INR level is calculated from the PT level.
- **aPTT (activated partial thromboplastin time):**
  - Normal: **30-40 seconds (not on Heparin)**
  - If the patient is on Heparin, the aPTT needs to be **1.5 to 2.5 times** the normal range.
- **PTT (partial thromboplastin time): 25-35 seconds**
- **D-dimer: <500 ng/mL FEU or <250 ng/mL DDU**
- **Fibrinogen:** 200-400 mg/dL

Lipid Panel

- **LDL (low density lipoprotein):** <100 mg/dL (want it LOW)
- **HDL (high density lipoprotein):** >60 mg/dL (want it HIGH)
- **Total Cholesterol:** <200 mg/dL
- **Triglycerides:** <150 mg/ dL

Assesses risk for cardiovascular disease.

Drug Levels

- **Digoxin:** 0.5-2 ng/mL
- **Acetaminophen:** 10-20 mcg/mL
- **Carbamazepine:** 4-10 mcg/mL
- **Dilantin:** 10-20 mcg/mL
- **Theophylline:** 10-20 mcg/mL
- **Salicylates:** 15-30 mg/dL
- **Phenobarbital:** 15-40 mcg/mL
- **Lithium:** 0.6-1.2 mEq/L
- **Valproic Acid:** 50-100 mcg/mL
- **Vancomycin**
  - **peak** 20-40 mcg/mL
  - **trough:** 10-20 mcg/mL

Cardiac Enzymes

- **Troponin I:** <0.04 ng/mL
- **Troponin T:** <0.01 ng/mL
- **CK:** 25-200 U/L
- **CK-MB:** 3-5% of total CK
- **Myoglobin:** 25 to 72 ng/mL
- **BNP:** <100 pg/ mL
- **NT-proBNP:**
  - <125 pg/mL <75 years old
  - <450 pg/mL >75 years old

Blood Gases

- **pH:** 7.35-7.45
- **PaCO2:** 35-45 mmHg
- **HCO3:** 22-26 mEq/L
- **PaO2:** 80-100 mmHg
- **O2 sat:** 95-100%

Diabetes Screening

HbA1c: hemoglobin A1c
- **<5.7%** (no diabetes)
- **5.7-6.4%** (prediabetes)
- **>6.5%** (diabetes)
- **<7%** (target for patients with diabetes)

Miscellaneous

- **GFR:** >90 mL/min/1.73m^2
- **Urine specific gravity:** 1.005 to 1.030
- **Ammonia:** 15-45 µ/dL
- **Amylase:** 40-140 U/L
- **Lipase:** 0-160 U/L

- **TSH:** 0.5-5 mIU/L
- **T3:** 80-180 ng/dL
- **T4:** 5-12 mcg/dL
- **Creatinine clearance test:** **females:** 85-130 & **males:** 90-140 mL/min

Chapter 1:
Fluid Compartments, Movement of Fluids and Solutes, & IV Fluid Types

Key Terms to Know:

FLUID COMPARTMENTS:

- **Extracellular**: outside the cell
  - **Intravascular**: fluid found inside the vessels (plasma)
  - **Interstitial**: fluid found between the cells
  - **Transcellular**: fluid found in the body cavities
- **Intracellular**: inside the cell

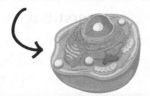

IV FLUID TYPES:

- **Colloids**: increases plasma volume by pulling water into intravascular space through oncotic pressure.
- **Hypertonic fluids**: crystalloid type IV fluids that have a higher osmolarity than the blood and will cause water to leave the intracellular space & move into extracellular space. This shrinks or dehydrates the cell.
- **Hypotonic fluids**: crystalloid type IV fluids that have a lower osmolarity than the blood and causes water to move from the extracellular space to the intracellular space. The cell will swell & can rupture.
- **Isotonic fluids**: crystalloid type IV fluids that have the same osmolarity as the blood and result in water equally transferring in and out of the cell.

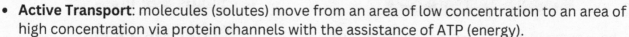

FLUID & SOLUTE MOVEMENT:

- **Active Transport**: molecules (solutes) move from an area of low concentration to an area of high concentration via protein channels with the assistance of ATP (energy).
- **Facilitated Diffusion**: molecules (solutes) move from an area of high concentration to an area of low concentration with assistance of proteins (no energy used).
- **Filtration**: the process that occurs when hydrostatic pressure pushes water and solutes out of the blood vessels (capillaries) into the interstitial space.
- **Hydrostatic Pressure**: the pressure or force of a fluid inside a restricted space. In other words, the "pushing" force of water when confided to a space.
- **Oncotic Pressure** (colloidal osmotic pressure): the "pulling" force on water created by proteins called albumin (a colloid).
- **Osmolarity**: the total concentration of solutes in a solution (per liter).
- **Osmosis**: water moves through a semipermeable membrane from an area of high water concentration to an area of low water concentration.
- **Osmotic Pressure**: pressure needed to stop movement of water due to osmosis.
- **Simple Diffusion**: molecules (solutes) move from an area of high concentration to an area of low concentration without the assistance of proteins (no energy used).
- **Solutes**: solids dissolved in a liquid (Ex. sodium and chloride are solutes in a bag of IV fluids).

Body Fluid Compartments:

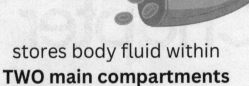

stores body fluid within **TWO main compartments**

Compartments

Intracellular:

- **Intra** means "inside"
- **cellular** means "the cell"
  This is called Intracellular **F**luid (**ICF**).

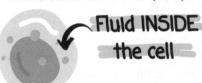

Fluid INSIDE the cell

- Most of our fluid is INSIDE the cell.
- Contains **2/3** of our body's water

Extracellular:

- **Extra** means "outside"
- **cellular** means "the cell"
  This is called **E**xtra**c**ellular **F**luid (**ECF**).
- Contains **1/3** of our body's water

Includes:

- **Intravascular:** fluid found inside vessels (plasma)
- **Interstitial:** fluid found between cells
- **Transcellular:** fluid found in body cavities (joints, spinal cord, etc.)

Function of Compartments

The compartments work together to maintain a **homeostatic environment** in the body by shifting around water, electrolytes, and other nutrients via different types of transport processes, such as **osmosis, diffusion, and active transport**.

Connecting the Dots

- Nurses **administer IV fluids** to the **intravascular compartment** to help expand it or shift fluids around in the compartments.
- **Osmosis** plays a role with helping correct fluid imbalances that can occur within the intracellular and extracellular spaces.

Movement of Fluids & Solutes

Water Movement

- **Osmosis:** water moves through a semipermeable membrane from an area of **high water concentration** to an area of **low water concentration**.

Solute Movement

- **Simple Diffusion:** molecules (solutes) move from an area of **high concentration** to an area of **low concentration (no energy used)**.
- **Facilitated Diffusion:** molecules (solutes) move from an area of **high concentration** to an area of **low concentration** with *assistance of proteins (no energy used)*.
- **Active Transport:** molecules (solutes) move from an area of **LOW concentration** to an area of **HIGH concentration** via protein channels with the assistance of **ATP (energy)**.

Movement of Fluids & Solutes
Cell Membrane & Transport:

movement can be through **passive** or **active** transport processes

Osmosis

Osmosis occurs when water moves from a fluid with a **low solute concentration** to a fluid with a **high solute concentration**. *In other words,* water moves from an area of high water concentration to an area of low water concentration.

Simplified:

- **Passive process:** no energy is required by the cell
- Water is drawn to the fluid with the **MOST solutes**.
  - **Solutes?** these are solids dissolved in a liquid...like sodium & chloride are solutes in a bag of IV fluids.

Solutes

Outside cell (extracellular)

Inside cell (intracellular)

Water moves this way

*high solutes, low water

*low solutes, high water

Osmotic pressure: pressure needed to stop movement of water due to osmosis

Semipermeable membrane: only allows **water** through (nothing else)

*In this example, there is **high osmotic pressure** inside the cell due to a high solute concentration.

Osmolarity is the total concentration of solutes in a solution (per liter).

IV fluids can have an **equal, high, or low osmolarity** when compared to the blood plasma.

↑osmolarity= **high** solutes, ↓water (**hypertonic**)

↓osmolarity= **low** solutes, ↑water (**hypotonic**)

Diffusion

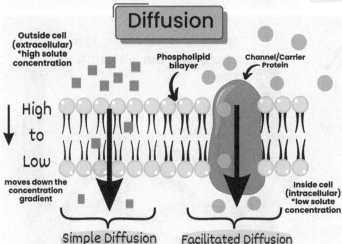

Outside cell (extracellular) *high solute concentration

Phospholipid bilayer

Channel/Carrier Protein

High to Low

moves down the concentration gradient

Inside cell (intracellular) *low solute concentration

Simple Diffusion

- Molecules (solutes) move from **high to low concentration**
- **Passive transport: NO energy**
- Cell's membrane (phospholipid bilayer) **ONLY** allows **TINY, non-charged molecules** like O2, CO2 etc. to go straight through.
- Diffusion occurs UNTIL **equilibrium is achieved** on the other side.

Facilitated Diffusion

- Molecules (solutes) move from **high to low concentration** through **special proteins.**
- **Why?** Proteins help transport big, charged, & polar molecules like glucose and ions into the cell that could NOT have went straight through phospholipid layer.
- **Passive transport: NO energy**

Active Transport

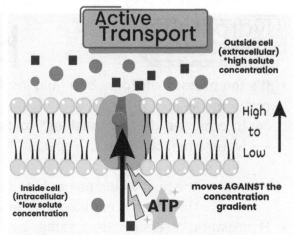

Outside cell (extracellular) *high solute concentration

High to Low

Inside cell (intracellular) *low solute concentration

ATP

moves AGAINST the concentration gradient

- Molecules (solutes) move from **low to high concentration** through special proteins with the assistance of **energy in the form of ATP.**
  - **Why energy?** Needs energy to go **against the concentration gradient**. This takes effort. If flowing down the concentration gradient (rather than against it) like with diffusion, no energy is needed, because it requires no effort.
- Example of this type of transport: **Sodium-potassium pump** (3 Na+ move out of cell, while 2 K+ move in cell)

4

Oncotic & Hydrostatic Pressure: "pull" and "push" effect on water across capillary wall

Oncotic Pressure

- Also called **colloidal osmotic pressure**
- It's the **"pulling"** force on water created by proteins called **albumin** (a colloid).
  - **Albumin** resides in the *blood plasma* & it is <u>too big</u> to pass through the capillary wall.
  - High concentrations of it hang out in the blood plasma (intravascular space).
    - This creates osmotic pressure and "pulls" water through a process known as osmosis.
    - <u>Result:</u> water stays in the vessel
- What happens if there **isn't enough albumin** (**hypoalbuminemia**)?
  - Water isn't "pulled" to stay in the vessel, but instead **leaves and goes into the interstitial space** & causes **SWELLING** in the tissues.
  - Causes: liver/kidney failure, major burns etc.

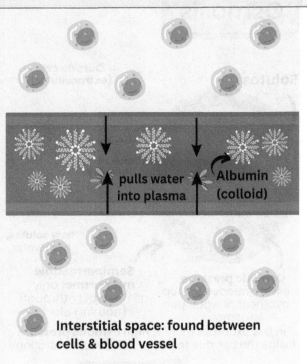

pulls water into plasma

Albumin (colloid)

Interstitial space: found between cells & blood vessel

Hydrostatic Pressure

- It's the pressure or force of a fluid inside a restricted space.
  - In other words, the **"pushing" force of water** when confided to a space.
    - Example of this in our body:
      - the fluid would be our blood and the space is our blood vessels
- Hydrostatic pressure is created by the **heart's contractions**.
- Hydrostatic pressure is **highest at the arterial end of the capillary** & **lowest at the venous end of the capillary**.
- This pressure pushes water and solutes out of the blood vessels (capillaries) into the interstitial space in a process known as **filtration**.

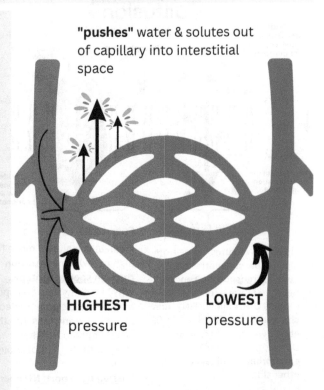

"pushes" water & solutes out of capillary into interstitial space

HIGHEST pressure

LOWEST pressure

IV Fluids: Colloids
Plasma Volume Expanders

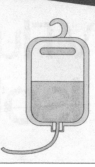

Function

How they Work?

- **Increases plasma volume** (intravascular space) by **"pulling"** water into this space through oncotic pressure (colloidal osmotic pressure).
- <u>How?</u>
  - Colloids are **very large molecules** that do **<u>NOT</u>** cross capillary wall but stay in the intravascular space. The **high number** (concentration) of these molecules cause an increase in oncotic pressure within the intravascular space, and **osmosis occurs**. The result is that **water is pulled into the intravascular space from interstitial space.** This increases the volume within this compartment.

Used for?

- Hypovolemic **shock**
- Severe **bleeding**
- **Burns**
- Hypo**albuminemia**

Types:

- **Natural**
  - Human albumin, fresh frozen plasma (FFP)
- **Synthetic:**
  - Hydroxyethyl starches (HES), Dextran, and Gelatin

Colloids vs Crystalloids

Colloids	Crystalloids
Includes **Albumin, Dextran, Hydroxyethyl starches (HES), Gelatin**	Includes **Hypotonic, Hypertonic, Isotonic** solutions
Large molecules that <u>**stay**</u> in intravascular space longer	**Small molecules** that <u>**don't stay**</u> too long in intravascular space
Fast at **expanding** intravascular space & amount administered equal to amount lost	**High amount** of **fluids needed** to equal amount lost **(overload: edema)**
Risks: allergic reaction, coagulation problems	**No** allergic reactions or coagulation problems
Cost More	**Cost Less** and easier to access

Nurse's Role

- **Assess allergies** & if any previous reactions to colloids in the past
  - Watch for gelatin allergy
- Monitor blood pressure, heart rate, oxygen saturation, respiratory rate, temperature **during administration per protocol**
- **Monitor for allergic reaction:** itching, hypotension, dyspnea, fever, etc.
  - **<u>STOP</u>** infusion, notify doctor
- Monitor for **bleeding problems:** increased PTT & PT level, low platelet count, hypotension, tachycardia
- **Monitor fluid status:** daily weights, strict I's and O's, **no** crackles, edema, s3 gallop

IV Fluids: Crystalloids Isotonic

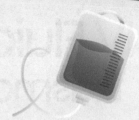

Function

How they Work?

- They have the **same osmolarity** as the blood (same concentration of solutes).
- **Result?** Water will **equally** transfer in and out of the cell
- Helps expand plasma (**intravascular**) which is part of the extracellular compartment

Benefits:

- Experiencing a **loss** of **ECF** due to vomiting & diarrhea
  - Needs some water, sodium & chloride back
- Hypovolemic **shock**
- **Burns**
- Prior to **surgery**
  - Losing ECF in surgery

Fluid Types

- 0.9% **Normal Saline**
- **Lactated Ringer's** Solution (LR)
- 5% **Dextrose in Water***

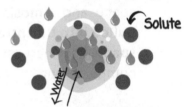

Equal solute concentration on **inside & outside** of cell
Result: cell stays the same

Nursing interventions

0.9% Normal Saline

- replaces **water, Na+, & CL-**
- The **ONLY** solution administered with **blood transfusion**

Watch for:

- **Fluid Overload-** putting too much fluid back into the extracellular compartment, especially in patients with **kidney and heart failure.**
- **Increase** in sodium and chloride levels

Lactated Ringer's

- contains **water, K+, Na+, CL-, Ca++, & lactate**
- The **lactate ↑ the blood's pH** by converting to *bicarb*. This can correct mild cases of **metabolic acidosis.**
- **Avoid** in liver disease (can't convert lactate to bicarb)
- **Avoid** in lactic acidosis (high amount of lactic acid)

Watch for:

- **Hyperkalemia risk,** especially in patients with renal failure

Dextrose 5% in Water

- replaces **water & dextrose**
- *Starts out as isotonic but turns into a **hypotonic** solution
- **Why?** Dextrose will be used by the body & what is left over is not very concentrated. It's **free water (low osmolarity),** so it becomes **hypotonic.**

Watch for:

- **Hyperglycemia** (not for fluid resuscitation due to this)

IV Fluids: Crystalloids Hypertonic

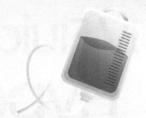

Function

How they Work?

- **Higher osmolarity** than the blood (higher concentration of solutes in the fluid)
- **Result?** Water will **leave** the **intracellular** space & **move** into **extracellular space**
- This **shrinks or dehydrates** the cell.

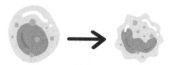

- Helps expand extracellular compartment

Benefits:

- **Severe hyponatremia**:
  - giving a hypertonic saline solution to the plasma will increase sodium blood levels.
- **Cerebral edema**: brain swelling

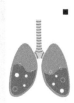
HELP!

  - **hypertonic solutions** will pull water from the brain cells and decrease swelling.

Fluid Types

- 3% Saline

- Dextrose 10% in water

- Dextrose 5% in 0.9% Normal Saline

- Dextrose 5% in 0.45% Normal Saline

How they work?

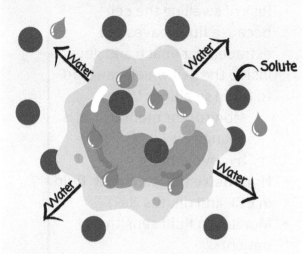

Water

Water

Solute

Water

Water

<u>HIGHER</u> solute concentration on **outside** of cell than the **inside**
Result: water moves from inside the cell to outside, and the **cell shrinks**

Nursing interventions

- Use **cautiously**
  - May overload the extracellular space, leading to **pulmonary edema** (fluid in the lungs) & **hypertension**
- May cause **hypernatremia**
- Always check with **facility's protocol** for how to properly administer these hypertonic solutions.

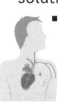

  - May need a **central line** for administration due to **extravasation risk**

8

IV Fluids: Crystalloids Hypotonic

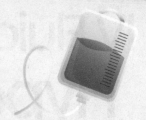

Function

How they Work?

- **Lower osmolarity** than the blood (lower concentration of solutes in the fluid)
- **Results?** Water **moves** from the **extracellular** space to the **intracellular** space.
- The cell will **swell** & can rupture.

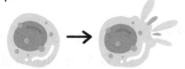

- Helps **replenish** water to the **inside of the cell**

Benefits:

- **Too much** solute concentration in the blood (**dilute** the concentration)
  - Hypernatremia
- Helps provide **free water to the kidneys** so they can excrete waste
- Prevent dehydration and **rehydrate** cells

Fluid Types

- 0.45% Saline (1/2 Normal Saline)

- 0.225% Saline

- 0.33% Saline

- 5% Dextrose in water **
  - **Classified as "isotonic" but works like hypotonic**

How they work?

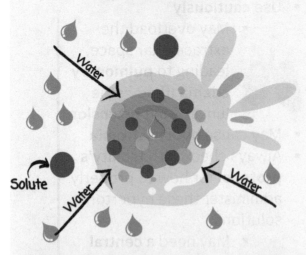

LOWER solute concentration on **outside** of cell than the **inside**
Result: water moves from outside of the cell to the inside, and the **cell swells and ruptures.**

Nursing interventions

- Risk of swelling the cell because fluid leaves the extracellular space and goes inside the cell which can lead to **brain swelling**:
  - Monitor for mental status changes
  - hypovolemia
- **Hyponatremia** (too much fluid in ECF and dilutes Na+)
- Monitor in fluid sensitive patients:
  - heart and renal failure (can't handle the extra free water)

Worksheet: IV Fluids

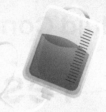

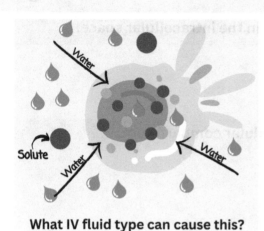

What IV fluid type can cause this?

_____

What IV fluid type can cause this?

_____

Match the IV fluid to its type:

- 3% Saline

- 0.225% Saline

- Lactated Ringer's

- Dextrose 10% in Water

- 0.9% Normal Saline

Hypotonic

Hypertonic

Isotonic

Fluid Compartments, Movements, & IV Solutions
Test Review

1. True or False: Most of the fluid in the body is found in the intracellular space.

A. True
B. False

2. Select all the fluid spaces that make up the extracellular compartment:

A. Transcellular
B. Extravascular
C. Intravascular (plasma)
D. Interstitial

3. What is the fluid compartment that surrounds the outside of the cells and plays a vital role in helping be a medium for electrolytes and other substances to move to and from the cell to the plasma?

A. Intracellular compartment
B. Interstitial compartment
C. Intravascular compartment
D. Transcellular compartment

4. What is the fluid compartment that is found inside the blood vessels?

A. Intracellular compartment
B. Interstitial compartment
C. Intravascular compartment
D. Transcellular compartment

5. What is the fluid compartment that is found in certain body cavities like the spinal cavity, heart, lungs, and joints?

A. Intracellular compartment
B. Interstitial compartment
C. Intravascular compartment
D. Transcellular compartment

11

Test Review

6. Which statement below is the most accurate about the process of osmosis?

A. Water will move from a solution with a higher solute concentration to a solution with a lower solute concentration.
B. Water and solutes will move from a lower water concentration solution to a higher water concentration solution.
C. Water will move from a lower solute concentration solution to a higher solute concentration solution.
D. Water will move from a fluid of a lower water concentration to a fluid of a higher water concentration.

7. True or False: Osmosis is an active transport process.

A. True
B. False

8. True or False: If a solution has a high concentration of solutes, it is considered to have a high osmolarity.

A. True
B. False

9. Which statements below best describe a hypotonic solution? Select all that apply:

A. It has a high osmolarity.
B. These fluid types have a lower amount of solutes in them compared to the blood plasma.
C. There is more water than solutes in these types of fluids.
D. These fluids can lead to cell shrinkage.

Test Review

10. What type of fluid below has a low osmolarity?

A. 0.9% Normal Saline
B. 3% Saline
C. Dextrose 5% in 0.9% Normal Saline
D. 0.45% Normal Saline

11. What is the only fluid type that can be administered with blood products?

A. Lactated Ringer's solution
B. 0.45% Normal Saline
C. 3% Saline
D. 0.9% Normal Saline

12. Which fluid below is considered an isotonic solution but works as a hypotonic solution?

A. Dextrose 5% in water
B. Lactated Ringer's solution
C. Dextrose 10% in water
D. 0.33% Normal Saline

13. Which patients below should not receive Lactated Ringer's solution? Select all that apply:

A. A patient with a mild case of metabolic acidosis
B. A pre-op patient scheduled for abdominal surgery
C. A patient experiencing hyperkalemia
D. A patient with liver failure

Fluid Compartments, Movements, & IV Solutions

Test Review

14. Which fluid type is MOST likely to cause hypernatremia along with fluid volume overload and requires close monitoring by the nurse during administration?

A. 0.45% Normal Saline
B. Dextrose 5% in water
C. 3% Saline
D. 0.225% Saline

15. Your patient is receiving 0.45% Normal Saline for hypernatremia. What finding requires you to stop the fluid and notify the doctor?

A. Decreasing sodium level
B. Increased urination
C. Confusion
D. Polydipsia

16. Which fluid below is NOT categorized as an isotonic fluid?

A. 0.9% Normal Saline
B. Lactated Ringer's solution (LR)
C. Dextrose 5% in water
D. Dextrose 5% in 0.45% Normal Saline

17. What type of solution below can be used to treat cerebral edema?

A. Isotonic
B. Hypertonic
C. Hypotonic

18. True or False: Lactated Ringer's Solution is first-line treatment for fluid resuscitation situations.

A. True
B. False

Fluid Compartments, Movements, & IV Solutions

Test Review

19. Which patient below is at risk for fluid volume overload while receive 0.9% Normal Saline?

A. A patient with hyponatremia
B. A patient experiencing dehydration
C. A patient with heart failure
D. A patient who is vomiting

20. What type of fluid can cause the cell the swell and rupture?

A. Isotonic
B. Hypertonic
C. Hypotonic

Use the Figures to answer the next questions: 21-31

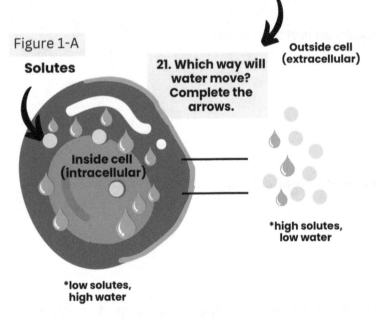

Figure 1-A

Solutes

21. Which way will water move? Complete the arrows.

Outside cell (extracellular)

Inside cell (intracellular)

*low solutes, high water

*high solutes, low water

Figure 1-A: Questions:

22. What type of fluid transport is illustrated ?

_____

23. Based on the water's movement, how will it affect the cell?

A. shrink   B. rupture   C. stay the same

24. What type of IV fluid can have this effect on the cell when administered?

A. hypotonic   B. hypertonic   C. isotonic

25. This fluid transport process is a type of active transport.

True   or   False

15

Fluid Compartments, Movements, & IV Solutions
Test Review

Figure 1-B

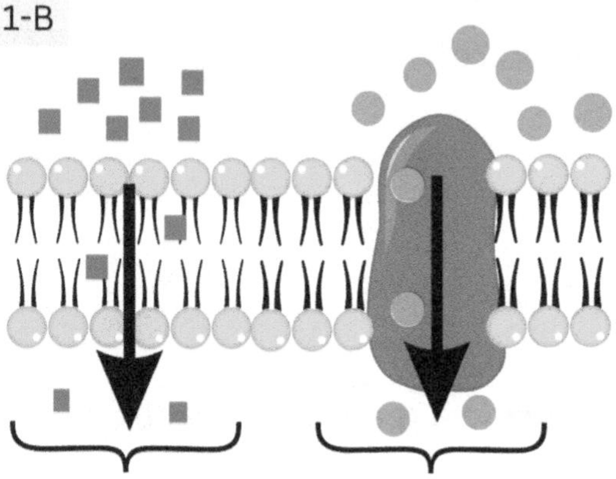

Figure 1-C

A. _____ B. _____

26. Label the types of transport above.

_____

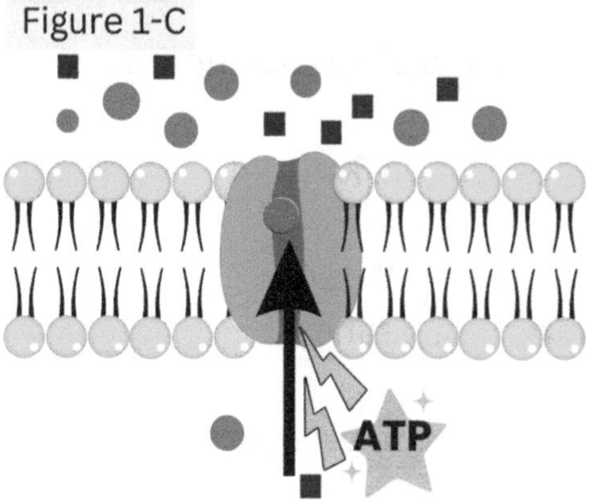

30. Label the type of transport above.

Figure 1-B: Questions:

27. Glucose and ions can only be transported via which type of transport?

        A   or   B

28. These types of transports move molecules down the concentration gradient?

      True   or   False

29. Are these transport processes known as active or passive transport?

      Active   or   Passive

Figure 1-C: Questions:

30. How does this type of transport move molecules?
    A. down the concentration gradient
    B. against the concentration gradient
    C. from high concentration to low concentration

31. Which statement is false about this type of transport?
    A. uses energy to move molecules
    B. uses proteins to assist in molecule movement
    C. is a passive form of transport
    D. is similar to the sodium-potassium pump

32. For each solution type, select if it is a characteristic for a colloid or crystalloid solution. Some characteristics may be for both solution types. Both columns will have at least one characteristic.

Characteristic	Colloids	Crystalloids
Includes Albumin, Dextran, Hydroxyethyl starches (HES), Gelatin	☐	☐
Expands plasma volume	☐	☐
High amount of fluid required to replace volume lost	☐	☐
Risk for allergic reaction	☐	☐

33. Which fluid type below increases oncotic pressure?

A. Normal Saline 0.9%
B. Dextran
C. Dextrose 5% in Water
D. 0.45% Normal Saline

34. _____ is the pressure or force of a fluid inside a restricted space.

A. Diffusion
B. Hydrostatic pressure
C. Oncotic pressure
D. Active transport

35. In what part of the capillary is hydrostatic pressure the highest?

A. Arterial end of the capillary
B. Venous end of the capillary
C. Arterial beginning of the capillary
D. Venous beginning of the capillary

36. What is a "pulling" force on water that is created by proteins like albumin?

A. Hydrostatic pressure
B. Filtration
C. Oncotic pressure
D. Facilitated diffusion

37. When hydrostatic pressure pushes water and solutes out of the blood vessels (capillaries) into the interstitial space, this is known as what process?

A. Reabsorption
B. Diffusion
C. Osmosis
D. Filtration

38. The nurse is administering Dextran IV. The patient develops severe itching and hypotension. What will the nurse do FIRST?

A. Administer an antihistamine
B. Notify the doctor
C. Slow down the infusion and reassess
D. Stop the infusion

 Answers for the questions are on the next page.

© Nurse Sarah (RegisteredNurseRN.com)

Worksheet: IV Fluids
Answers & Rationales

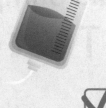

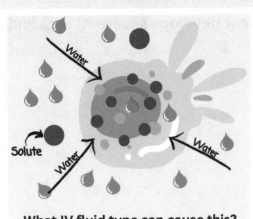

What IV fluid type can cause this?

Hypotonic

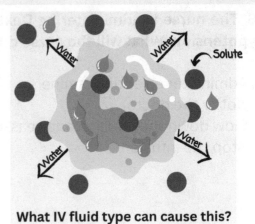

What IV fluid type can cause this?

Hypertonic

Match the IV fluid to its type:

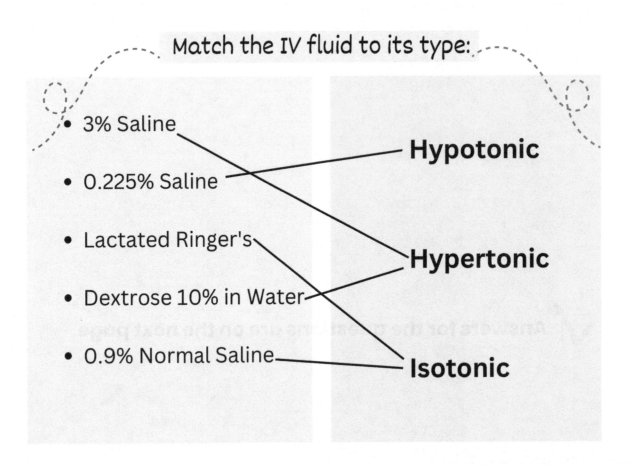

- 3% Saline
- 0.225% Saline
- Lactated Ringer's
- Dextrose 10% in Water
- 0.9% Normal Saline

Hypotonic

Hypertonic

Isotonic

Fluid Compartments & IV Solutions
Answers & Rationales ✓

1. The answer is TRUE. The intracellular space is the space inside of the cell. The fluid in it accounts for 2/3 of our body water. Therefore, most of our fluid is inside the cell.

2. The answers are A, C, and D. The interstitial, intravascular, and transcellular fluid compartments make up the extracellular compartment.

3. The answer is B: interstitial compartment

4. The answer is C: intravascular compartment

5. The answer is D: transcellular compartment

6. The answer is C. Osmosis is the movement of water from a fluid of higher water concentration to a fluid of lower water concentration. In other words, water will move from a lower solute concentration fluid to a higher solute concentration fluid.

7. The answer is FALSE. Osmosis is a passive type of transport process.

8. The answer is TRUE.

9. The answers are B and C. Hypotonic solutions have a lower osmolarity than the blood plasma (lower concentration of solutes in the fluid). Osmosis will cause water to move from the extracellular space to the intracellular and swell the cell, which can rupture.

10. The answer is D. 0.45% Normal Saline is a hypotonic solution. It contains a lower concentration of solutes compared to the blood plasma. Due to this, it will cause water to move from the extracellular space to the intracellular space, which could swell the cell leading to possible rupture.

11. The answer is D. 0.9% Normal Saline is the ONLY fluid that can be administered with blood products.

12. The answer is A. Dextrose 5% in water (D5W) starts out as an isotonic solution, but

☑️

ends up working as a hypotonic solution. This occurs because once the dextrose in the solution is used by the body (metabolized), there is only free water left over, which has a low osmolarity and acts as a hypotonic solution.

13. The answers are C and D. Lactated Ringer's solution (LR) contains water, potassium, sodium, chloride, calcium, and lactate. Patients who are experiencing hyperkalemia (high potassium level) should not receive this solution since it already has potassium in it. In addition, a patient with liver failure is not a candidate for LR because it contains lactate. The liver is responsible for converting lactate to bicarbonate. When the liver is failing, this conversion process cannot happen, which can lead to the buildup of lactate.

14. The answer is C. 3% Saline is a hypertonic solution and contains a concentrated amount of sodium. It will cause fluid to leave the intracellular space and enter the extracellular space. This could lead to fluid volume overload and requires very close monitoring by the nurse. The other solutions listed here are hypotonic.

15. The answer is C: confusion. 0.45% Normal saline is a hypotonic solution. It can be used to treat hypernatremia (it lowers the sodium levels in the blood). This fluid causes osmosis to move water from the extracellular space to the intracellular space. If too much is moved to the intracellular space, cell swelling can present. Signs of this include mental status changes like confusion. Therefore, the nurse would want to hold the fluid and notify the doctor for further orders. Polydipsia is excessive thirst, which presents with hypernatremia. Increased urination and a decreasing sodium level are expected.

16. The answer is D: Dextrose 5% in 0.45% Normal Saline. This is a hypertonic solution. Dextrose 5% in water is considered isotonic, but once administered it becomes hypotonic (it categorized as an isotonic fluid).

17. The answer is B. Cerebral edema is swelling of the brain. Hypertonic solutions dehydrate the cell which is helpful with cerebral edema.

Fluid Compartments & IV Solutions
Answers & Rationales

18. The answer is FALSE. LR contains glucose which can increase the blood glucose and is not first-line treatment for fluid resuscitation situations.

19. The answer is C. In cases of heart failure, the heart is too weak to pump fluid out of the heart. This can lead the body to become overwhelmed with fluid. Patients who are experiencing heart or kidney failure are at risk for fluid volume overload when receiving fluids.

20. The answer is C.

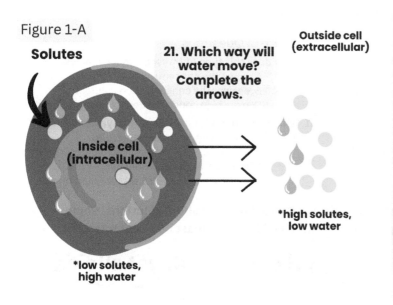

Figure 1-A

Solutes

21. Which way will water move? Complete the arrows.

Outside cell (extracellular)

Inside cell (intracellular)

*high solutes, low water

*low solutes, high water

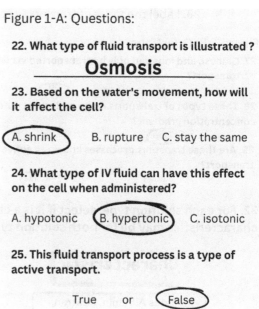

Figure 1-A: Questions:

22. What type of fluid transport is illustrated ?
Osmosis

23. Based on the water's movement, how will it affect the cell?

A. shrink   B. rupture   C. stay the same

24. What type of IV fluid can have this effect on the cell when administered?

A. hypotonic   B. hypertonic   C. isotonic

25. This fluid transport process is a type of active transport.

True   or   False

Fluid Compartments & IV Solutions
Answers & Rationales

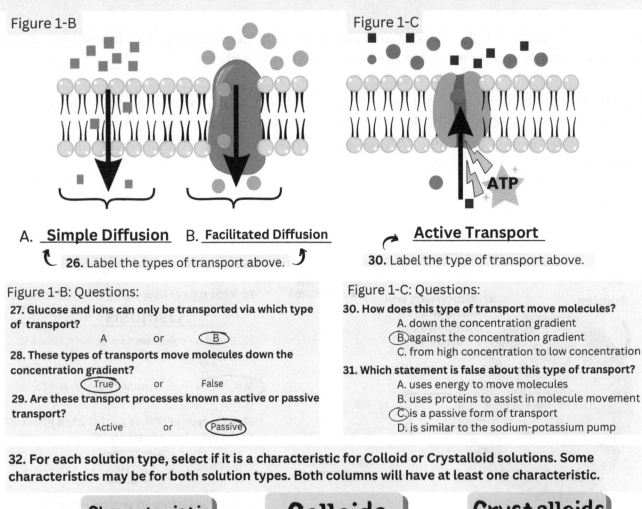

Figure 1-B

A. **Simple Diffusion**   B. **Facilitated Diffusion**

↳ **26.** Label the types of transport above. ↲

Figure 1-C

Active Transport

↳ **30.** Label the type of transport above.

Figure 1-B: Questions:

27. Glucose and ions can only be transported via which type of transport?

A   or   (B)

28. These types of transports move molecules down the concentration gradient?

(True)   or   False

29. Are these transport processes known as active or passive transport?

Active   or   (Passive)

Figure 1-C: Questions:

30. How does this type of transport move molecules?
   A. down the concentration gradient
   (B.) against the concentration gradient
   C. from high concentration to low concentration

31. Which statement is false about this type of transport?
   A. uses energy to move molecules
   B. uses proteins to assist in molecule movement
   (C.) is a passive form of transport
   D. is similar to the sodium-potassium pump

32. For each solution type, select if it is a characteristic for Colloid or Crystalloid solutions. Some characteristics may be for both solution types. Both columns will have at least one characteristic.

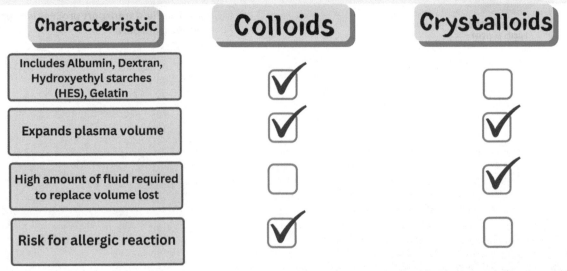

Characteristic	Colloids	Crystalloids
Includes Albumin, Dextran, Hydroxyethyl starches (HES), Gelatin	✓	
Expands plasma volume	✓	✓
High amount of fluid required to replace volume lost		✓
Risk for allergic reaction	✓	

Answers & Rationales

33. The answer is B: Dextran. This is a type of synthetic colloidal solution. It has large molecules that stay in the intravascular system longer, creating oncotic pressure (also called colloidal osmotic pressure).

34. The answer is B: Hydrostatic pressure.

35. The answer is A: arterial end of the capillary. This is where the hydrostatic pressure is the highest, and as blood flow continues, the pressure decreases. Hydrostatic pressure is the lowest at the venous end of the capillary.

36. The answer is C: oncotic pressure.

37. The answer is D: filtration.

38. The answer is D: stop the infusion. Dextran is a synthetic colloid and can cause an allergic reaction. First, the nurse should stop the infusion and then proceed with notifying the doctor.

Chapter 2:

Fluid Balance:
Hormones & Body Systems

Key Terms to Know:

HORMONES:

- **Aldosterone**: causes the kidneys to keep sodium and water (also waste potassium) to help increase blood volume.
- **Antidiuretic hormone (ADH)**: causes the kidneys to reabsorb water and increase fluid volume.
- **Atrial natriuretic peptide (ANP)**: hormone released by the heart cells due to atrial wall stretching.
- **Brain natriuretic peptide (BNP)**: hormone released by the heart cells due to ventricle wall stretching.

BODY SYSTEMS:

- **Hypothalamus**: makes antidiuretic hormone (ADH).
- **Osmoreceptors:** found in the hypothalamus and are sensitive to high plasma osmolarity, which stimulates the thirst mechanism.
- **Posterior Pituitary Gland**: stores and secretes antidiuretic hormone (ADH).
- **Renin-Angiotensin-Aldosterone System (RAAS)**: purpose is to correct a low blood pressure by increasing blood volume
- **Thirst Mechanism**: purpose is to correct a fluid volume deficit & high osmolality in plasma.

Hormones in Fluid Regulation

Antidiuretic Hormone

- Also called **ADH**
- Made in the **hypothalamus**
- Stored & released by the **posterior pituitary gland**
- When fluid levels drop & plasma osmolality increases:
  - **Osmoreceptors** in the hypothalamus respond & cause ADH to be released
  - **RAAS** creates **angiotensin II,** which influences ADH & causes it to be released
- ADH causes distal convoluted tubule & collecting duct in nephron to **REABSORB WATER**
- **Purpose**: increases fluid volume in blood

Summary:

Aldosterone

- Made & released by the **adrenal cortex**
- Release of aldosterone is controlled by the **Renin-Angiotensin-Aldosterone System (RAAS)**
- **Purpose:** causes kidneys to **keep sodium (Na+) & water** rather than excreting it into urine. However, it does cause the **wasting of K+**.
  - increases fluid volume in blood

Natriuretic Peptides

- **Atrial natriuretic peptide (ANP):** hormone released by the heart cells due to **atrial wall stretching**

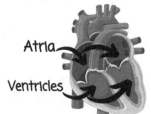

Atria

Ventricles

- **Brain natriuretic peptide (BNP):** hormone released by the heart cells due to **ventricle wall stretching**.
  - These hormones **work against angiotensin II.**
  - **Stops effects** of aldosterone, ADH, and renin

RAAS

- Known as the **R**enin-**A**ngiotensin-**A**ldosterone **S**ystem
- **Its purpose** is to correct a low blood pressure by increasing blood volume.

Sequence of RAAS:

1. Juxtaglomerular cells release **renin**.
2. Liver **activates angiotensinogen**, which turns into **angiotensin I**.
3. ACE (**A**ngiotensin-**C**onverting **E**nzyme) turns angiotensin I into **angiotensin II**.
4. **Angiotensin II** causes:
   a. major **vasoconstriction**
   b. release of **aldosterone** & **ADH**
   c. stimulates thirst mechanism

Thirst Mechanism

- **Its purpose** is to correct a fluid volume deficit & high osmolality in plasma.
  - High osmolality of plasma means low fluid in plasma and high solutes (mainly sodium).

Sequence of Thirst Mechanism:

1. **Osmoreceptors** in hypothalamus respond & cause **ADH to be released** by the posterior pituitary gland.
2. **ADH** causes the distal convoluted tubule & collect duct in the nephron of the kidneys to **put water back into the blood** rather than the urine.
3. **Water** stays in the blood & **increases fluid volume & helps normalize plasma osmolality.**

Renin-Angiotensin-Aldosterone System

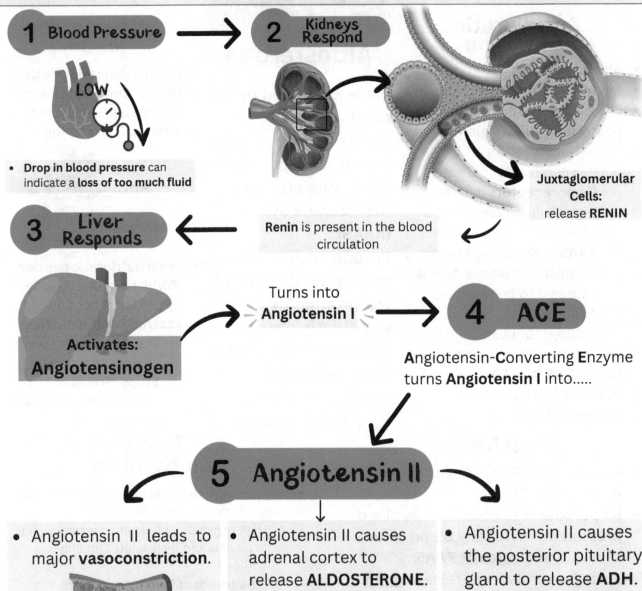

1 Blood Pressure → **2** Kidneys Respond

LOW

- **Drop in blood pressure** can indicate a **loss of too much fluid**

Juxtaglomerular Cells: release **RENIN**

3 Liver Responds ← **Renin** is present in the blood circulation

Activates: **Angiotensinogen**

Turns into **Angiotensin I** → **4** ACE

Angiotensin-Converting Enzyme turns **Angiotensin I** into.....

5 Angiotensin II

- Angiotensin II leads to major **vasoconstriction**.
- Constricting blood flow to the kidneys limits its ability to excrete water.
  - Keeps more water in blood to increase fluid volume & blood pressure

- Angiotensin II causes adrenal cortex to release **ALDOSTERONE**.

  - Leads the kidneys to keep sodium and water in blood
  - Decreases urination

- Angiotensin II causes the posterior pituitary gland to release **ADH**.
  - Leads the kidneys to keep water and increases blood volume
  - **Stimulates thirst mechanism**

27

© Nurse Sarah (RegisteredNurseRN.com)

Mechanism of Thirst

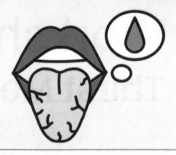

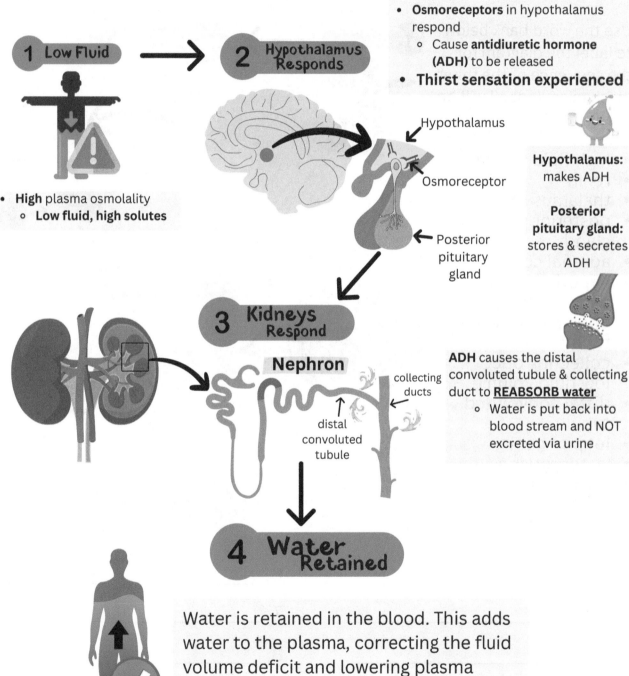

1 Low Fluid

- **High** plasma osmolality
  - **Low fluid, high solutes**

2 Hypothalamus Responds

- **Osmoreceptors** in hypothalamus respond
  - Cause **antidiuretic hormone (ADH)** to be released
- **Thirst sensation experienced**

Hypothalamus

Osmoreceptor

Posterior pituitary gland

Hypothalamus: makes ADH

Posterior pituitary gland: stores & secretes ADH

3 Kidneys Respond

Nephron

collecting ducts

distal convoluted tubule

ADH causes the distal convoluted tubule & collecting duct to **REABSORB water**
  - Water is put back into blood stream and NOT excreted via urine

4 Water Retained

Water is retained in the blood. This adds water to the plasma, correcting the fluid volume deficit and lowering plasma osmolality to normal.

Worksheet:
Thirst Mechanism Sequence

Use the word bank below to label the diagram for the sequence of the thirst mechanism (not all will be used).

- high fluid volume
- renin
- thalamus responds
- posterior pituitary gland
- adrenal cortex
- hypothalamus
- osmoreceptors
- proximal convoluted tubule
- collecting duct
- low fluid volume
- distal convoluted tubule
- loop of henle
- water retained
- hypothalamus responds
- kidneys responds

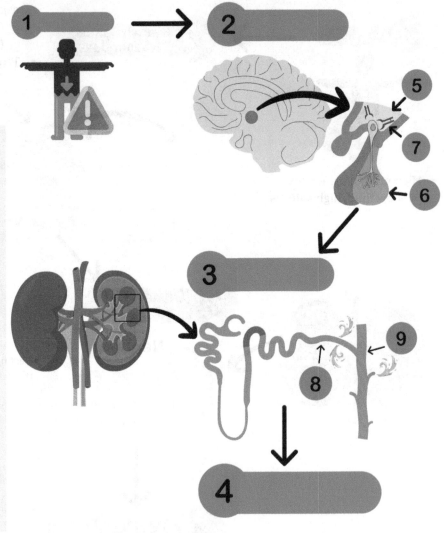

1. _____

2. _____

3. _____

4. _____

5. _____

6. _____

7. _____

8. _____

9. _____

29

Worksheet:
Renin-Aldosterone-Angiotensin System

Use the word bank below to label the diagram for the sequence of RAAS (renin-aldosterone-angiotensin system). Not all options will be used.

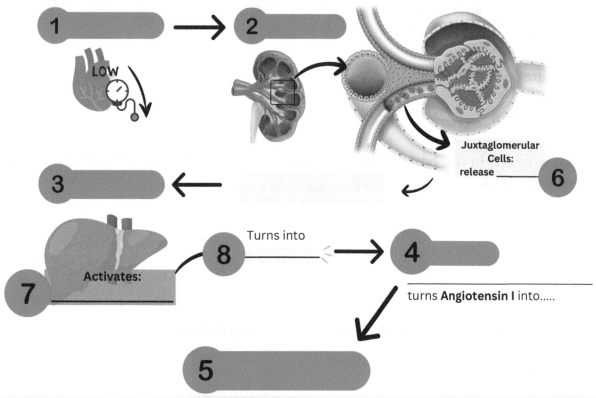

- renin
- aldosterone
- antidiuretic hormone
- angiotensin I

- blood pressure
- kidneys respond
- angiotensin II
- atrial natriuretic peptide

- liver responds
- angiotensinogen
- ACE (angiotensin-converting enzyme)

1. _____

2. _____

3. _____

4. _____

5. _____

6. _____

7. _____

8. _____

Hormones in Fluid Regulation Test Review

1. What does the juxtaglomerular cells release as part of the Renin-Angiotensin-Aldosterone System?

A. Aldosterone
B. Antidiuretic hormone
C. Renin
D. Angiotensin II

2. What organ(s) in the body activates angiotensinogen when it senses the presence of renin in the circulation?

A. Kidney
B. Heart
C. Lungs
D. Liver

3. What substance does angiotensinogen turn into in RAAS?

A. Angiotensin II
B. Renin
C. Aldosterone
D. Angiotensin I

4. What is the role of ACE (Angiotensin-Converting Enzyme)?

A. Turns renin into angiotensin II
B. Turns angiotensin I into angiotensin II
C. Turns angiotensin I into aldosterone
D. Turns angiotensin I into renin

Hormones in Fluid Regulation Test Review

5. Select all the roles of Angiotensin II:

A. Vasoconstriction
B. Vasodilation
C. Release renin
D. Lead to the release of aldosterone
E. Lead to the release of ADH
F. Stimulate thirst mechanism
G. Decrease blood volume

6. What structure in the body makes antidiuretic hormone (ADH)?

A. Kidneys
B. Posterior pituitary gland
C. Hypothalamus
D. Adrenal cortex

7. When a patient is low on fluid or has a high plasma osmolality, what structure in the body responds to this issue first in the thirst mechanism?

A. Hypothalamus
B. Thalamus
C. Adrenal glands
D. Kidneys

8. True or False: Osmoreceptors in the hypothalamus cause antidiuretic hormone to be released.

9. What structure stores and secretes ADH?

A. Kidneys
B. Posterior pituitary gland
C. Hypothalamus
D. Adrenal cortex

Hormones in Fluid Regulation Test Review

10. What parts of the nephron in the kidney respond to antidiuretic hormone (ADH)? Select all that apply:

A. Loop of Henle
B. Bowman's capsule
C. Distal convoluted tubule
D. Proximal convoluted tubule
E. Collecting duct

11. What is the purpose of antidiuretic hormone (ADH)?

A. Reabsorb sodium and water to increase fluid volume in the blood
B. Reabsorb water to increase blood volume
C. Cause vasoconstriction to increase blood volume
D. Waste sodium and water to increase blood volume

12. What hormone is released by the heart cells due to atrial wall stretching?

A. ANP
B. BNP
C. Aldosterone
D. Antidiuretic hormone

13. What hormone is released by the heart cells due to ventricle wall stretching?

A. ANP
B. BNP
C. Aldosterone
D. Antidiuretic hormone

14. What hormones work against the effects of Angiotensin II? Select all that apply:

A. Aldosterone
B. Atrial natriuretic peptide
C. Brain natriuretic peptide
D. Renin

 Answers for the questions are on the next page.

33

Hormones in Fluid Regulation Answers and Rationales ☑

1. low fluid volume
2. hypothalamus responds
3. kidneys responds
4. water retained
5. hypothalamus
6. posterior pituitary gland
7. osmoreceptors
8. distal convoluted tubule
9. collecting duct

Answers to RAAS Diagram:

1. blood pressure
2. kidneys respond
3. liver responds
4. ACE (angiotensin-converting enzyme)
5. angiotensin II
6. renin
7. angiotensinogen
8. angiotensin I

Answers to Questions:

1. The answer is C: renin. Juxtaglomerular cells respond to a low blood pressure and released renin.

2. The answer is D: liver. The liver activates angiotensinogen when it senses the presence of renin in the circulation.

3. The answer is D: angiotensin I. Angiotensinogen turns into angiotensin I.

4. The answer is B: turns angiotensin I into angiotensin II. ACE, Angiotensin-Converting Enzyme, has an important role for converting angiotensin I into angiotensin II.

Hormones in Fluid Regulation Answers and Rationales

5. The answers are A, D, E, and F. Angiotensin II will cause: vasoconstriction, lead to the release of aldosterone and ADH, and stimulate the thirst mechanism. It will INCREASE blood volume (not decrease) because it has a goal of increasing blood pressure.

6. The answer is C: hypothalamus. This structure makes ADH, but it is stored and secreted by the posterior pituitary gland.

7. The answer is A: hypothalamus

8. The answer is TRUE.

9. The answer is B: posterior pituitary gland. This structure stores and secretes ADH. ADH is made in the hypothalamus.

10. The answers are C and E. These structures of the nephron are affected by ADH and reabsorb water back into the blood stream. Therefore, water goes back into the plasma and helps increase blood volume.

11. The answer is B: reabsorb water to increase blood volume. This is the purpose of antidiuretic hormone.

12. The answer is A: ANP. This stands for atrial natriuretic peptide.

13. The answer is B: BNP. This stands for brain natriuretic peptide and is released by heart cells due to ventricle wall stretching.

14. The answers are B and C. These are natriuretic peptides that work against angiotensin II and stop the effects of aldosterone, ADH, and renin.

Chapter 3: Electrolytes

Key Terms to Know:

IMBALANCES:

- **Electrolytes**: these are substances that once dissolved in water (hence our blood), produce an electrical charge. This helps with electrical signaling in the body and other important processes.
- **Hypernatremia**: high sodium level in blood >145 mEq/L
- **Hyponatremia**: low sodium level in blood <135 mEq/L
- **Hyperchloremia**: high chloride level in blood >105 mEq/L
- **Hypochloremia**: low chloride level in blood <95 mEq/L
- **Hyperkalemia**: high potassium in blood >5 mEq/L
- **Hypokalemia**: low potassium in blood <3.5 mEq/L
- **Hypercalcemia**: high calcium in the blood >10.5 mg/dL
- **Hypocalcemia**: low calcium in the blood <8.5 mg/dL
- **Hyperphosphatemia**: high phosphate in the blood >4.5 mg/dL
- **Hypophosphatemia**: low phosphate in the blood <2.5 mg/dL
- **Hypermagnesemia**: high magnesium in the blood >2.5 mg/dL
- **Hypomagnesemia**: low magnesium in the blood <1.5 mg/dL

PREFIXES & SUFFIXES:

calc: calcium   **chlor**: chloride   **emia**: blood

kal: potassium   **magnes**: magnesium   **natr**: sodium

hyper: high or increased   **hypo**: low or decreased

phosphat: phosphate

Electrolytes &
Their Relationships

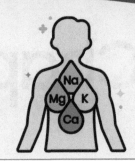

What are Electrolytes?

These are substances that once dissolved in water (hence our blood), produce an **electrical charge**. This **helps with electrical signaling** in the body and other important processes like:

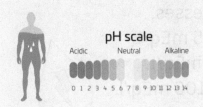

pH scale

Acidic   Neutral   Alkaline

0 1 2 3 4 5 6 7 8 9 10 11 12 13 14

- Contraction of **muscles**
- Sending **nerve impulses**
- Creating **bones**
- Balancing the **fluids**
- Maintaining **acid-base balance**

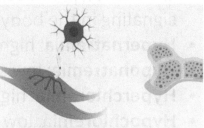

- Electrolytes must be **BALANCED!**
- **Imbalanced** electrolytes create **problems** in the body
- Imbalances can range from **mild to severe**

Nurse's Role:
- assessing for signs & symptoms
- monitoring lab results
- administering treatments
- providing education

Electrolyte Relationships:

Inverse:

electrolytes increase or decrease in **opposite directions**

↓ Magnesium = ↑ Phosphate

↑ Sodium = ↓ Potassium

↑ Calcium = ↓ Phosphate

Direct:

electrolytes increase or decrease in **same direction**

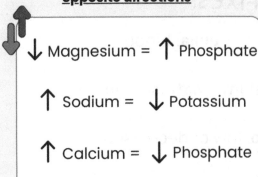

↓ Magnesium = ↓ Calcium

↓ Magnesium = ↓ Potassium

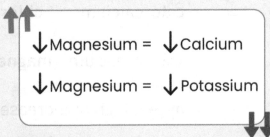

Vitamin

D helps increase absorption of calcium & phosphate:

Low Vitamin D = Low Ca+ and Phos.

Function of Electrolytes

Sodium

- Normal level is **135-145 mEq/L**
- Abbreviated as **Na+**
- Mainly hangs out in the **extracellular compartment**
- Helps regulate water inside & outside of the cell
- Plays a role in **muscle contraction & transmission of nerve impulses**
- **Vital Fact:** When levels of **Na+ drop** in the blood, it affects the cells because suddenly water starts to rush inside the cell. This causes the cell to **SWELL.**
  - On the flip side, when too much Na+ is in the blood, water from inside the cell starts to leave and the cell **SHRINKS.**

Chloride

- Normal level is **95-105 mEq/L**
- Abbreviated as **Cl-**
- Role with **acid-base & fluid balance**
- **Cl- & Na+** hang out and work together.
  - If Na+ low, *usually* Cl- too
- Makes up **hydrochloric acid**
- **Kidneys help maintain** Cl- levels by excreting it in the urine.
  - Also excreted through sweat & gut juices
- If imbalanced (**especially high**), it is usually due to a **kidney problem**.

Potassium

- Normal level is **3.5-5 mEq/L**
- Abbreviated as **K+**
- Mainly hangs out in the **intracellular compartment**
- Responsible for **nerve impulse** conduction & **muscle contraction**
- K+ helps with fluid balance like Na+, especially **inside the cell.**
- **K+ & Na+** have an **inverse relationship.**
  - Na+ increases, potassium decreases

Calcium

- Normal level is **8.5-10.5 mg/dL**
- Abbreviated as **Ca++**
- **Absorbed** in the **GI system**
- **Stored** in the **bones**
- Levels maintained w/ the help of:
  - **Vitamin D:** absorption of Ca++
  - **Parathyroid hormone:** produced by the parathyroid gland
    - causes bones to release Ca++ in blood to **increase levels**
  - **Calcitonin:** produced by the thyroid gland
    - does the opposite of parathyroid hormone to decrease **Ca++ levels**
- Ca++ & phosphate have an **inverse relationship**
  - **Calcium ↑ = ↓ Phosphate**
- Ca++ & Mg have a **direct relationship**

Phosphate

- Normal level is **2.5-4.5 mg/dL**
- Abbreviated as **PO4**
- Role with **acid-base & fluid balance**
- **Stored** in bones & absorbed from food via the **GI system**
- **Excreted** via **kidneys**
  - **High phosphate level** is usually a **sign kidneys** are failing.
- Plays a role with:
  - **building bones/teeth**
  - **nerve/muscle function**
- **Parathyroid gland** plays a role in the regulation of phosphate
- **Vitamin D** helps w/ absorption
- Has an **inverse relationship** with **Ca++ and Mg**

Magnesium

- Normal level is **1.5-2.5 mg/dL**
- Abbreviated as **Mg**
- Mainly hangs out in the **intracellular compartment**
- **Absorbed** in the **gut** (small intestine)
- **Excreted** via **kidneys**
- Plays a role with:
  - **nerve transmission**
  - **muscle relaxation**
  - **how vessels work to maintain blood pressure**
  - **heart muscle contraction process**
- **Direct relationship** with K+: (decrease Mg = decrease K+)
- Mg helps **make parathyroid hormone,** which increases Ca++.
  - if Mg low, it will decrease Ca++
- **Inverse relationship** with PO4: (decrease Mg = increase PO4)

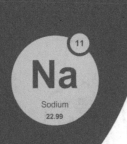

Na 11
Sodium
22.99

Hypernatremia
High sodium level in blood

More than 145 mEq/L
(Normal level 135-145 mEq/L)

Causes:

- ## Medications

  Corticosteroids

  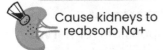 Cause kidneys to reabsorb Na+

  Hypertonic Solutions

  3% Normal Saline
  5% Normal Saline

- ## Cushing's syndrome

  ↘ **High cortisol causes Na+ retention** but K+ loss

- ## Primary Hyperaldosteronism
  (Conn's syndrome)

  HYPER aldosterone production = Na+ retention

- ## Not Drinking Enough Water

  Increases Na+ concentration in the blood

- ## Losing too much Water

  🔹Vomiting 🔹Diarrhea
  🔹Burns 🔹Sweating
  🔹Diabetes Insipidus

- ## High intake of Sodium

Signs & Symptoms:

Remember: "No **FRIED** foods for you, *too much sodium!*"

Fatigue

Restless Confused

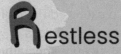
Central nervous system changes ←

Increased reflexes
(progress to seizure & coma)

Extreme **THIRST** BIG sign

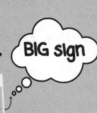

Dry mouth & skin

w/ **decreased urine output**

Nursing interventions

- ## RESTRICT Sodium Intake

  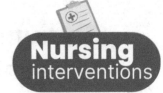
  X Foods HIGH in SALT
  bacon   butter
  canned   hot dogs
  foods   cheese
  lunch meat

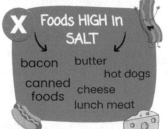
⚠ Keep patient **SAFE**
(patient may be **confused** and **restless**)

- ## IV Solutions may be ordered

- **Isotonic**
  ✓ 5% Dextrose
- **Hypotonic**
  ✓ 0.45% Normal Saline

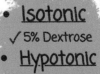

Give Hypotonic solutions **SLOWLY**: can cause brain swelling

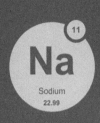

Na ¹¹
Sodium
22.99

Hyponatremia
Low sodium level in blood

Less than 135 mEq/L
(Normal level 135-145 mEq/L)

Causes:

- **Euvolemic**
  hyponatremia:
  body water increases, but Na+ stays the same

  SIADH
  (**S**yndrome of **I**nappropriate **A**nti**D**iuretic **H**ormone)

  High ADH = ↑ Body Water
  Adrenal insufficiency (Addison's Disease)
  Hypothyroidism

  Low Thyroid Hormone

- **Hypovolemic**
  hyponatremia:
  body water and **Na+ loss**
  ↳ greatest loss

  ✓Vomiting, Diarrhea, GI suction
  ✓Diuretic therapy
  ✓Burns   ✓Sweating

- **Hypervolemic**
  hyponatremia:
  body water and **Na+ increases**

  HELP!
  ✓Heart Failure
  ✓Renal Failure
  ✓Liver Failure

  ↳ *water increase is more than the Na+ increase*
  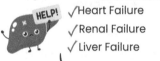

Signs & Symptoms:

Remember: "Salt Loss"

Seizures & Stupor

Abdominal cramping

Lethargic

Tendon reflexes ↓

Loss of urine & appetite

Orthostatic hypotension

Shallow respirations
LATE due to skeletal muscle weakness

Spasms of muscles

40

Nursing interventions

- **INCREASE oral** Sodium Intake
  ✓ Foods HIGH in SALT
  bacon   butter
  canned   hot dogs
  foods   cheese
           lunch meat

  Doctor may prescribe **Sodium Tablets** in some cases

- **SIADH** the cause?

  <u>Demeclocycline</u>
  tetracycline family: works as an **ADH ANTAGONISTS**
  Don't give w/ foods like DAIRY or ANTACIDS
  FLUID RESTRICTION!

- **Hypovolemic** hyponatremia?

  IV Sodium Chloride Infusions to restore Na+ & fluid

- **Hypervolemic** hyponatremia?

- **RESTRICT** Fluids
- **Diuretics** to remove excess water...this helps *concentrate* Na+
- **Renal Failure?** Dialysis

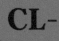

CL-

Hyperchloremia
High chloride level in blood

More than 105 mEq/L
(Normal level 95-105 mEq/L)

Causes:

- **High intake of Sodium**

Hypertonic Solutions

Too much **IV Saline**

High Sodium Intake

- **Loss of Fluid**

Not drinking enough water

Losing water
↳ **Diabetes insipidus:** losing too much **urine**

Loss of Bicarbonate through diarrhea
↳ **Metabolic acidosis**
- Causes a **decrease in bicarbonate levels**
- **Elevates** CL- levels
- **Bicarb & CL-** have an **opposite relationship**

- **Hyperaldosteronism**

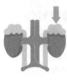

Too much aldosterone: retain sodium along with fluid and excrete potassium

- **Corticosteroids**
cause **kidneys to retain** Na & CL-

Signs & Symptoms:

Note: **S & S of hyperchloremia** tend to be associated with whatever is causing the high level rather than the level being high itself.

So you want to look at what is causing the high level.

The **S & S** will be like the ones found in **HYPERnatremia & acidosis:**

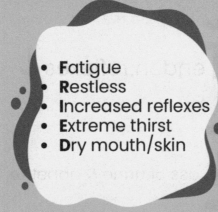

- **F**atigue
- **R**estless
- **I**ncreased reflexes
- **E**xtreme thirst
- **D**ry mouth/skin

Others due to acidosis:

- Increased deep respirations
  - **Kussmaul breathing**
- Tachycardia
- Confused
- Vomiting
- Nausea

Nursing interventions

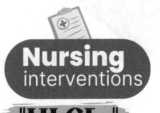

"HI CL-"

Hold sodium chloride **infusions**. Prevents further increase of CL-.

Limit intake of sodium & chloride rich foods. Needs **low sodium diet**.

Instead **Lactated Ringers (LR)** may be used to help **decrease chloride**.

The **lactate** in the **LR solution** turns into **bicarb** which helps <u>increase bicarb levels & lower chloride</u>. Remember, bicarb and chloride have an opposite relationship.

Helpful w/ **treating metabolic acidosis**. Bicarb increases blood pH & makes blood less acidotic.

Collect **intake & output, vital signs**, daily **weights**

Labs to monitor:

- **Chloride**
- **Sodium**
- **Bicarbonate (HCO3-)**
- **Potassium: hyperkalemia** can occur if acidosis presents.

This is because **potassium leaves the cell** and moves into the extracellular fluid (hence the blood) in exchange for hydrogen ions.

41

CL-

Hypochloremia
Low chloride level in blood

Less than 95 mEq/L
(Normal level 95-105 mEq/L)

Causes:

• Loss of CL-

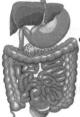

GI tract
- NG Suction
- Emesis
- Ileostomy

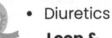

Renal
- Diuretics
- **Loop & Thiazides** waste CL- in urine

Cystic Fibrosis

- **Too much CL-** loss in sweat

• Metabolic Alkalosis

- Causes an **increase in bicarbonate levels**
- **Lowers** CL- levels
- **Bicarb & CL-** have an **opposite relationship**

• Fluid Overload

- dilutes ECF & lowers CL-as in **Heart Failure**
- **Too much ADH** (SIADH): retain water dilutes CL- & Na+

Signs & Symptoms:

Note: **S & S of hypochloremia** tend to be associated with whatever is **causing the low level** rather than the level being low itself.

So you want to look at what is causing the low level to identify the signs and symptoms.

The **S & S** will be like the ones found in **HYPOnatremia:**

Seizures	**L**oss of urine
Abdominal cramps	**O**rthostatic
Lethargic	**S**hallow Resp.
Tendon reflexes	**S**pasms

Others:
- Dehydration
  - **increased** heart rate
  - **decreased** blood pressure
  - **fever**
- Vomiting
- Diarrhea

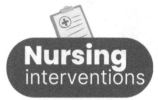

Nursing interventions
"LOSS"

Look at **SODIUM level** & assess for S&S of **HYPOnatremia**

Remember "**SALT LOSS**"

In addition:
- Assess **neuro status due to confusion** from brain swelling
- Initiate **seizure** precautions
- Monitor **respiratory** status
- **I**ntake & **O**utput
- **V**ital **S**igns
- **Weights**

Other **LABS** to monitor:

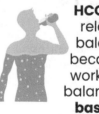

- **HIGH** bicarb (HCO3-)
- **LOW** potassium (K+) especially if this is due to **metabolic alkalosis**

  HCO3- & K+ are related to the balance of CL- because they all work together to balance the **acid-base system** & our **fluid balance in the body.**

Saline IV to replace CL-

Sources of CL- rich foods

- table salt
- tomatoes
- olives

- seafood
- processed meat
- canned food

Hyperkalemia
High potassium level in blood

More than 5 mEq/L
(Normal level 3.5-5 mEq/L)

Causes:

- ### Medications

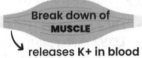
Potassium-sparing **DIURETICS**

Example: **Sp**ironolactone
↳ **Sp**ares K+ in kidneys

ACE Inhibitors

Example: Lisino**pril**
↳ Lowers **ALDOSTERONE**
(decreases K+ excretion)

- ### Burns
releases K+ into blood

- ### Rhabdomyolysis

Break down of **MUSCLE**
↓
releases K+ in blood

- ### Addison's Disease

low aldosterone causes kidneys to waste sodium but **ADD** (keeps) potassium

- ### Renal Failure

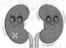

- ### Excessive Intake of K+

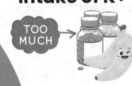
TOO MUCH

Signs & Symptoms:

High potassium levels are very dangerous and can lead to **DEATH!**

Decreased Heart Rate

EARLY: muscle twitching
Ascending weakness
Starts in legs & progresses UP to arms
T
E

Arrhythmias

Ventricular Fibrillation **(LATE)**
- **TALL, peaked T waves**
- Flat P wave
- Prolonged PR interval
- Wide QRS complex

Tummy Trouble

Increased movement of food through GI system
(Nausea, Vomiting, Diarrhea)

Hypotension

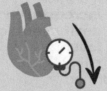

Nursing interventions

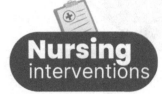

- **Watch ECG**, respiratory rate, neuro, GI, & renal system.

- **STOP** IV infusion of potassium & hold any PO supplements

- Initiate **K+ Restricted Diet**

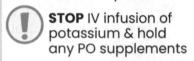
Remember K+ rich foods

- May need **Dialysis**

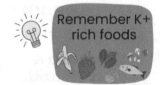

Administer Medications
to Decrease K+ Level

Diuretics: waste K+ in urine
↳ **Loop Diuretics & Thiazides**

Kayexalate: helps **ex**crete K+ by promoting GI sodium absorption
↳ Given PO or via enema

Hypertonic Solutions of Dextrose & **Regular** Insulin
↳ helps **pull K+ into cell** to drop blood levels

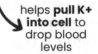

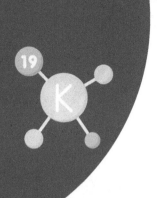

Hypokalemia
Low potassium level in blood

Less than 3.5 mEq/L
(Normal level 3.5-5 mEq/L)

Causes:

- ### Medications

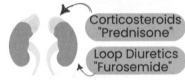

Corticosteroids "Prednisone"

Loop Diuretics "Furosemide"

These meds cause the kidneys to **WASTE** K+

- ### Too much insulin

Moves K+ into cell from the blood, which **depletes** the blood level

- ### Cushing's Syndrome

↑cortisol causes kidneys to keep Na+ & **waste K+**

- ### Loss from GI

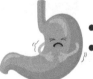

- Emesis
- Suction

- ### Starvation

Not consuming enough potassium

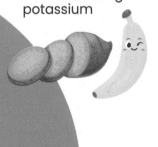

Signs & Symptoms:

We have a **low potassium level,** so everything is going to be _SLOW_ & _LOW._

7 L's

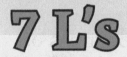

1. Lethargy
2. Low, shallow respirations
3. Lethal cardiac rhythms
4. Lots of voiding
5. Leg cramps
6. Limp muscles
7. Low blood pressure & heart rate

Nursing interventions

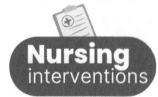

- **Watch ECG**, respiratory rate, neuro, GI, & renal system.
- **Monitor for low** Magnesium (hard to increase K+ if Mg is low)

Glucose, Sodium, & Calcium can be affected too

- **Administer oral K+** supplements per order

Usually for levels 2.5-3.5
- Give w/ food due to GI upset

- **Potassium IV infusion** for levels less than 2.5

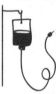

NEVER give Potassium via:
- IV push
- Intramuscular
- Subcutaneous

- Infuse at ordered rate (has to be given slowly)
- Can cause **phlebitis**

If Hypokalemia presenting:
- don't give loop diuretics or thiazides...waste more K+
- don't give Digoxin: **Digoxin Toxicity**
- Educate patient on **foods HIGH** in "**Potassium**"

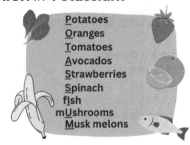

Potatoes
Oranges
Tomatoes
Avocados
Strawberries
Spinach
f**I**sh
m**U**shrooms
Musk melons

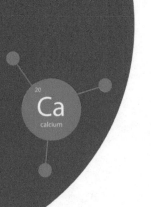

Hypercalcemia
High calcium level in blood

More than 10.5 mg/dL
(Normal level 8.5-10.5 mg/dL)

Causes:

• Medications

Thiazide Diuretics

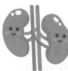

increases **renal reabsorption** of **calcium**

Example: Hydrochlorothiazide

Lithium:

affects the parathyroid & **increases PTH**

This increases calcium levels.

Too Much Vitamin D and/or Calcium Supplements

• Hyperactive Parathyroid Gland

→ **too much PTH** produced causes **increase in calcium** blood levels

• Bone Cancer

breaks down the bone which leaks calcium into the blood & **increases** levels

Signs & Symptoms:

Remember: A major finding will be that body systems are

"WEAK".

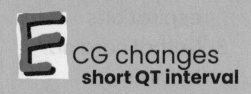
Weakness of **muscle**

ECG changes **short QT interval**

Absent reflexes ↓
Altered mental status
Abdominal distention (Constipation)

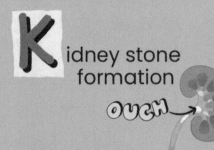
Kidney stone formation
OUCH →

Nursing interventions

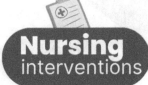

• Mild cases

- **Safe** from falls or injury
- **Hydration** to prevent kidney stone formation

S & S of Kidney Stone?

- Flank or abdominal **pain**
- **Urge** to void
- **Pain** w/ voiding
- **Decreased** urine flow ↓

Strain urine

- **Limit foods** high in calcium

• Moderate cases

Administer **calcium reabsorption inhibitors:**
- calcitonin
- bisphosphonates
- prostaglandins synthase inhibitors

• Severe cases
Dialysis

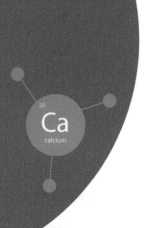

Hypocalcemia
Low calcium level in blood

Less than 8.5 mg/dL
(Normal level 8.5-10.5 mg/dL)

Causes:

- **Medications**

Bisphosphonates:
makes **bones stronger** by **decreasing the release of calcium from the bones into** the blood
RESULT: Bones release less calcium into blood
Example: Alendronate

Aminoglycosides:
group of antibiotics that cause kidneys to **waste calcium**
Example: Amikacin & Tobramycin

Anticonvulsants:
alters **Vitamin D levels**
Example: Phenobarbital & Phenytoin

- **Thyroid or Parathyroid Surgery**

Damage to the parathyroid
Always assess for HYPOcalcemia post-op

- **Low Calcium Intake**
Lactose intolerant

- **Low Vitamin D levels**

- **Kidney Disease**

Signs & Symptoms:

Remember: Muscles and nerves will → **CRAMP**

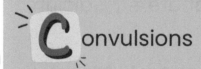
Convulsions

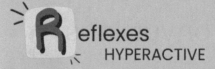
Reflexes
HYPERACTIVE

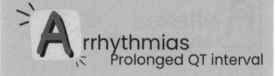
Arrhythmias
Prolonged QT interval

Muscle spasms in calves or feet (tetany)

Positive Signs of:

Trousseau
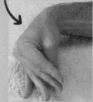

Chvostek
Tap on **Masseter Muscle:** facial muscle will **TWITCH**

46

Nursing interventions

- **Encourage** foods **HIGH** in calcium:

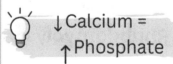
Foods HIGH in ↓ Calcium ↓
milk   yogurt
rhubarb   cheese
sardines   tofu

- **IV calcium** may be ordered

Example:
Calcium Gluconate

- Give slowly
- Monitor ECG
- Assess for infiltration or phlebitis
- Best to give via central line

- **Oral Calcium w/ Vitamin D**

↓ Calcium = ↑ Phosphate

⚠ **Patient safety risks:**

Bone fractures, seizures, laryngeal spasms

© Nurse Sarah (RegisteredNurseRN.com)

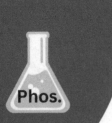

Phos.

Hyperphosphatemia
High phosphate level in blood

More than 4.5 mg/dL
(Normal level 2.5-4.5 mg/dL)

Causes:

- Over usage of **PHOSPHATE**-based **LAXATIVES**

  Example: Fleet Enema

- Too many **Vitamin D supplements**

  ↘ Increases **Renal** reabsorption & **GI** absorption

- **Hypoparathyroidism**

  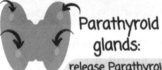

  Parathyroid glands:
  release <u>Parathyroid Hormone (PTH)</u>

  Normally, PTH inhibits kidney reabsorption of phosphate, **BUT** when <u>**underactive**</u>, it causes phosphate to be reabsorbed by the kidneys...**increasing levels.**

- **Rhabdomyolysis**

  break down of muscle occurs and **myoglobin** enters bloodstream

  ↓ leads to renal failure & the decrease of PHOSPHATE excretion

Signs & Symptoms:

Remember:

$$\uparrow Phosphate = \downarrow Calcium$$
$$\downarrow Phosphate = \uparrow Calcium$$

S & S present as **HYPOcalcemia**

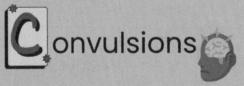
Convulsions

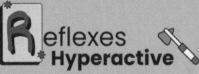
Reflexes **Hyperactive**

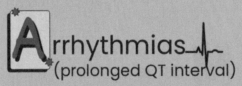
Arrhythmias
(prolonged QT interval)

Muscles spasms
in calves & feet (tetany)

Pruritus (itching)
associated w/ renal failure

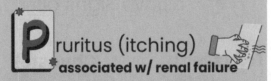
Signs of: Chvostek's & Trousseau

Nursing interventions

- **DECREASE foods** High in Phos.

  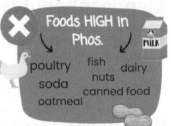
  ❌ Foods HIGH in Phos.
  poultry · fish · dairy
  soda · nuts
  oatmeal · canned food

- Administer **Phosphate-Binding** Meds

  <u>Calcium Acetate</u>
  Causes Phosphate to be **excreted through the stool**
  ✓ **Give w/ meals or right after eating**

- AVOID **Phosphate** containing Meds

  Laxatives or Enema

- **Prep for Dialysis** if in renal failure

  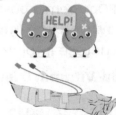

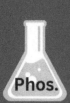

Phos.

Hypophosphatemia
Low phosphate level in blood

Less than 2.5 mg/dL
(Normal level 2.5-4.5 mg/dL)

Causes:

- **Long-term usage of Aluminum-based antacids**

  blocks the **absorption** of *phosphate* by the intestines

- **Overactive Parathyroid Gland**

  Parathyroid glands:
  release Parathyroid Hormone (PTH)

  Parathyroid gland plays a role in maintaining **calcium and phosphate** levels. It normally *inhibits reabsorption* of phosphate by the kidneys.

  Overactive Parathyroid = Kidneys quit reabsorbing PHOSPHATE

- **Starvation or refeeding syndrome**

  - Reintroduction of food **increases the release of insulin.**
  - **Phosphate** is needed by the body's cells to change glucose into energy.
  - This majorly **decreases phosphate levels.**

- **Low Vitamin D**

- **Burns**

  Moves Phosphate intracellularly

- **Alcoholism**

  malnutrition & poor diet

Signs & Symptoms:

S & S present when levels are **severely LOW** (not mildly)

Bone pain & fractures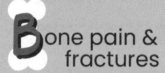

Osteomalacia
(results in leg bowing & short stature in children)

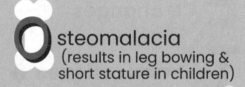

Neuro changes
confusion, irritability, seizures

Erythrocyte destruction
(red blood cells destroyed leading to **hemolytic anemia**)

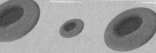

Nursing interventions

- **Increase foods** HIGH in Phos. **but** LOW in Calcium

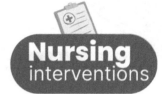

  ✓ Foods HIGH in Phos.
  pork   beef
  fish   organ meat
  poultry

- Administer **oral phosphorus w/ Vitamin D**

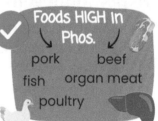

  Remember **Vitamin D** helps with *absorbing phosphate*

  If Phos. Level < 1 mg/dL:
  IV phosphorous may be ordered

  ⭐ Monitor for:
  Low Calcium & High Phosphate Levels

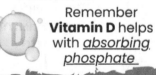

Assess **BUN & Creatinine** *before* giving **phosphorous**

If renal failure is present, kidneys can't clear phosphate....**increases levels.**

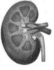 Ensure patient safety due to risk of Bone Fractures

Hypermagnesemia
High magnesium level in blood

More than 2.5 mg/dL
(Normal level 1.5-2.5 mg/dL)

Causes:

Not very common but it can happen in cases of:

- **Hypomagnesemia**

  when **trying to correct a low Mg level**
  (Too much Mg given)

- **Preeclampsia treatment**

  Receiving **Magnesium Sulfate**

  Toxicity: Decreased or ABSENT **D**eep **T**endon **R**eflexe**s**

- **Impaired Kidney Function**

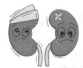

  kidneys **fail to excrete** Mg

  INCREASING LEVELS

Signs & Symptoms:

Note: You will typically **only see symptoms in severe cases** of hypermagnesemia. In mild cases the patient may be asymptomatic.

HYPERmagnesemia leads body systems to be **"LETHARGIC"**.

(opposite for hypomagnesemia, where body systems are excited)

Lethargy

ECG changes
wide QRS, long PR & QT interval

Tendon reflexes ⬇

Hypotension

Arrhythmias
bradycardia, third-degree heart block

Red & hot face
Flushing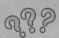

Gastrointestinal:
nausea & vomiting

Impaired breathing
due to muscle weakness

Confusion ⁇⁇

Nursing interventions

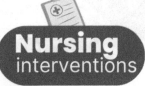

- **Monitor ECG** rhythm for changes

- Prevention: Avoid administering antacids & laxatives containing **Magnesium** to patients in RENAL FAILURE.

❌ **LIMIT Mg rich foods**
  nuts   green leafy vegs
  cauliflower   potatoes
  legumes   avocados

- **Loop or Thiazide Diuretics** may be ordered to help waste Mg by the kidneys.

  NOT for pts. in renal failure

- Assess for **hyper**magnesemia when treating low Mg levels w/ **Magnesium Sulfate**

   Diminished or Absent DTRs

- **IV calcium** may be ordered to reverse respiratory & cardiac effects of high Mg levels

49

Mg

Hypomagnesemia
Low magnesium level in blood

Less than 1.5 mg/dL
(Normal level 1.5–2.5 mg/dL)

Causes:

- **Medications**

Thiazide & Loop Diuretics

cause the **kidneys to waste Mg**

Proton Pump Inhibitors (PPIs)

decreases absorption of Mg via intestines

- **Not absorbing or consuming enough Mg**

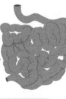
  - Starvation
  - Alcoholism
  - Bowel Disorders: **Crohn's & Ulcerative colitis**

- **Type 2 Diabetes**

causes the **kidneys to waste Mg in urine**

Signs & Symptoms:

Remember: When Mg is **too low** to calm things down, **excitability** will be occur and systems are going to **TWITCH!**

(opposite for **hyper**magnesemia)

Trousseau & **Chvostek Sign**

Low Mg causes **hypocalcemia** due to affecting the **Parathyroid gland**

Weakness

Increased reflexes

Torsades de Pointes & tetany → LETHAL

Calcium & potassium: LOW

Low Mg causes **kidneys to waste potassium**

Hypertension

Nursing interventions

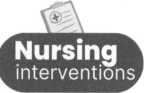

- **Monitor ECG** rhythm for changes
- **Monitor** for Hypo**kal**emia & Hypo**calc**emia

- May need **Potassium supplements** if hypo**kal**emia present

 difficult to correct low Mg level if **K+ is low too**

- May need **Calcium supplements** if hypo**calc**emia present

 Oral or **IV** Calcium

- **IV Magnesium Sulfate** to replace Mg

Toxicity → Assess for **DECREASED** OR **ABSENT D**eep **T**endon **R**eflexe**s**

- **Increase Mg rich foods**
  nuts   green leafy vegs
  cauliflower   potatoes
   legumes   avocados

- **Seizure Precautions**

Electrolytes
Test Review

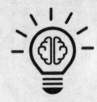

1. Magnesium is absorbed by what system of the body?

A. GI
B. Hepatic
C. Renal
D. Lymphatic

2. A patient is presenting with a low magnesium level of 1.3 mg/dL. Which of the following is NOT a sign or symptom of this condition?

A. Hypertension
B. Torsades de pointes
C. Positive Trousseau's sign
D. Absent deep tendon reflexes

3. Which patient below is at MOST risk for hypermagnesemia?

A. A patient with alcoholism.
B. A patient taking a proton-pump inhibitor.
C. A patient suffering from Crohn's disease.
D. A patient receiving IV magnesium sulfate via an infusion.

4. Stimulation of the facial nerve via the masseter muscle that causes twitching of the nose/lips in hypocalcemia is known as?

A. Trousseau's sign
B. Chvostek's sign
C. Homan's sign
D. Goodell's sign

5. A patient is presenting with hypocalcemia and has a calcium level of 7.2 mg/dL. What sign below is associated with this lab value?

A. None, this is a normal calcium level
B. Shortened ST segment
C. Hypoactive bowel sounds
D. Prolonged QT interval on the EKG

51

Electrolytes
Test Review

6. An EKG shows a shortened QT interval. Which lab value below would be associated with this finding?

A. Calcium level of 8 mg/dL
B. Calcium level of 12 mg/dL
C. Calcium level of 8.7 mg/dL
D. Calcium level of 9.2 mg/dL

7. Which patient below is considered hypernatremic?

A. A patient with a sodium level of 155 mEq/L
B. A patient with a sodium level of 145 mEq/L
C. A patient with a sodium level of 120 mEq/L
D. A patient with a sodium level of 136 mEq/L

8. A patient has a low sodium level of 119 mEq/L. Which of the following is NOT related to this finding?

A. Oversecretion of ADH (antidiuretic hormone)
B. Low-salt diet
C. Inadequate water intake
D. Hypotonic fluid infusion (overload)

9. A patient's blood test shows they have a critically low parathyroid hormone (PTH). What effect would this have on phosphate and calcium levels in the blood?

A. Phosphate levels high, calcium levels low
B. Phosphate and calcium levels high
C. Phosphate and calcium levels low
D. Phosphate levels low, calcium levels high

Electrolytes
Test Review

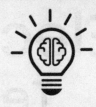

10. Which of the following would you NOT expect to see with a low phosphate level of 1.2 mg/dL?

A. Positive Trousseau's sign
B. Anemia
C. Confusion
D. Osteomalacia

11. A patient has a low potassium level of 1.5 mEq/L. Which of the following is NOT typically a sign with this condition?

A. None, this is a normal potassium level
B. Decreased respirations
C. Decreased deep tendon reflexes
D. Tall T-waves

12. Which patient is at risk for hyperkalemia?

A. Patient taking a loop diuretic
B. Patient with Cushing's syndrome
C. Patient with Addison's disease
D. Patient with nasogastric suction

13. Which of the following does chloride NOT play a role in?

A. Digestion
B. Acid-base balance
C. Fluid balance
D. Bone health

Electrolytes
Test Review

14. A patient has a low chloride level of 70 mEq/L. Which condition below can cause this type of level?

A. Heart failure
B. Cystic fibrosis
C. Metabolic acidosis
D. Hypertonic fluids

15. A positive Trousseau's sign is associated with which of the following electrolyte imbalances? Select all that apply:

A. Hyperkalemia
B. Hypocalcemia
C. Hyperphosphatemia
D. Hyponatremia

16. A patient has a low sodium level. Select the most appropriate nursing intervention for this patient:

A. Limit fluid intake to 3 liters per day
B. Administer hypotonic solutions
C. Offer the patient a deli sandwich, potato chips, and dill pickles
D. Encourage the patient to consume oranges, avocados, and fish

17. Your patient has a low potassium level of 2 mEq/L. Which order received by the doctor would require the nurse to obtain clarification?

A. Administer Furosemide IV
B. Administer IV potassium solution
C. Administer Spironolactone by mouth
D. Hold dose of Digoxin

Electrolytes
Test Review

18. A patient is experiencing torsades de pointes on the ECG. The nurse assesses the patient's current lab work. Which electrolyte imbalance is associated with this type of rhythm?

A. Hyperkalemia
B. Hypermagnesemia
C. Hypomagnesemia
D. Hypokalemia

19. A patient is post-op from a thyroidectomy. The nurse would immediately report what sign and symptom?

A. Flushing
B. Tetany
C. Muscle weakness
D. Constipation

20. Parathyroid hormone (PTH) _____ calcium levels, and calcitonin _____ calcium levels.

A. Decreases; increases
B. Decreases; decreases
C. Increases; decreases
D. Increases; increases

21. What type of IV fluids may be prescribed for hypernatremia?

A. 3% Saline
B. Dextrose 5% in Normal Saline
C. Dextrose 10% in Water
D. 0.45% Normal Saline

Electrolytes
Test Review

22. What are some roles chloride has in the body? Select all that apply:

A. Creating hydrochloric acid
B. Bone and teeth health
C. Blood clotting
D. Acid-base balance

23. True or False: Hypertonic fluids can lead to hypochloremia.

A. True
B. False

24. Which intervention below should be avoided in cases of severe hyperchloremia?

A. Administering IV Normal Saline infusion
B. Administering IV Lactated Ringers solution
C. Restricting the patient's consumption of deli meats
D. Monitoring intake and output

25. Hyperkalemia could lead to what type of ECG change?

A. Prolonged QT interval
B. Short PR interval
C. Tall, peaked t-wave waves
D. Missing QRS complexes

Electrolytes
Test Review

26. The doctor prescribes the patient to take Kayexalate. As the nurse, you know this medication is prescribed to do what?

A. Decrease potassium blood levels
B. Increase potassium blood levels
C. Increase magnesium levels
D. Decrease magnesium levels

27. What hormone is from the thyroid gland and plays a role with decreasing calcium levels?

A. Parathyroid hormone (PTH)
B. Calcitonin
C. Vitamin D
D. Aldosterone

28. The doctor orders calcium acetate (Phoslo) for your patient. The nurse knows this medication is used to treat?

A. Low phosphate levels
B. High phosphate levels
C. High sodium levels
D. Low sodium levels

29. The nurse is administering IV magnesium sulfate for hypomagnesemia. What symptoms below demonstrate possible magnesium toxicity?

A. Constipation
B. Increased deep tendon reflexes
C. Decreased deep tendon reflexes
D. Positive Chvostek's sign

Electrolytes
Answers & Rationales

1. The answer is A: GI

2. The answer is D: Absent deep tendon reflexes

3. The answer is D: A patient receiving IV magnesium sulfate via infusion

4. The answer is B: Chvostek's Sign

5. The answer is D: Prolonged QT interval on the EKG

6. The answer is B: Calcium level of 12 mg/dL. A high calcium level can cause a shortened QT interval.

7. The answer is A: A patient with a sodium level of 155 mEq/L

8. The answer is C: Inadequate water intake

9. The answer is A: Phosphate levels high, calcium levels low

10. The answer is A: Positive Trousseau's sign

11. The answer is D: Tall t-waves (this presents with <u>hyper</u>kalemia). Hyper means high, so remember it will have high or tall t-waves.

12. The answer is C: Addison's disease

13. The answer is D: Bone health

14. The answer is B: Cystic fibrosis

15. The answers are B and C. Hypocalcemia and hyperphosphatemia are associated with a positive Trousseau's sign. Remember that calcium and phosphate have an opposite relationship.

Electrolytes
Answers & Rationales

16. The answer is C. These food options are high in sodium, which is what the patient needs. The patient needs a fluid restriction (3 L is too much fluid per day and not restricted enough), and hypotonic solutions provide too much free water to the intravascular compartment (further diluting the sodium level). Option D are foods high in potassium.

17. The answer is A. Furosemide is a loop diuretic that wastes potassium and will further lower the level.

18. The answer is C: Hypomagnesemia

19. The answer is B. Hypocalcemia is a risk with thyroidectomy because it can damage the structures that help maintain calcium levels. The nurse would want to report tetany (muscle spasms), positive Trousseau's and Chvostek's sign, convulsions, hyperactive reflexes, and arrhythmias, as these are some of the signs and symptoms of hypocalcemia.

20. The answer is C.

21. The answer is D. 0.45% Normal Saline is a hypotonic solution, which can be used for hypernatremia. In addition, isotonic solutions can be used.

22. The answers are A and D. Chloride is needed to make hydrochloric acid, which plays a role in food digestion. In addition, it plays a role with acid-base balance in the body.

23. The answer is FALSE. Hypertonic fluids have a high osmolarity (high amount of solutes). Solutions like 3% saline could lead to hypernatermia and hypercholoremia.

24. The answer is A. Administering normal saline infusions would further increase chloride levels and should be avoided.

25. The answer is C. Hyperkalemia can lead to tall peaked t-waves, prolonged PR interval, ST depression, and wide QRS complex.

Electrolytes
Answers & Rationales

26. The answer is A. Kayexalate is sometimes ordered and given PO or via enema. This drug promotes GI sodium absorption, which causes potassium excretion.

27. The answer is B. Calcitionin decreases calcium blood levels, while PTH increases the levels.

28. The answer is B. Calcium acetate (Phoslo) is a phosphate-binding drug that works on the GI system and causes phosphorus to be excreted through the stool. Be sure to give with meals or right after the patient eats a meal.

29. The answer is C. Magnesium toxicity presents with a decrease in deep tendon reflexes. The nurse should be checking DTRs routinely during an IV infusion of magnesium sulfate.

Chapter 4:
Acid-Base Imbalances

Key Terms to Know:

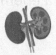 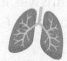

IMBALANCES:

- **Respiratory acidosis**: decreased lung ventilation that results in high carbon dioxide level & low blood pH.
- **Respiratory alkalosis**: increased lung ventilation that results in low carbon dioxide level & high blood pH.
- **Metabolic acidosis**: increase of acids in the body that results in a low blood pH and low bicarbonate level.
- **Metabolic alkalosis**: decrease of acid or increase of bicarbonate in the body that results in a high blood pH.

REMEMBER THESE LABS:

- **Respiratory Acidosis:**
Blood pH: <7.35
PaCO2: >45 mmHg
HCO3-: Normal or elevated (>26 mmHg)

- **Respiratory Alkalosis:**
Blood pH: >7.45
PaCO2: <35 mmHg
HCO3-: Normal or decreased (<22 mmHg)

- **Metabolic Acidosis:**
Blood pH: <7.35
HCO3-: <22 mmHg
PaCO2: Normal or decreased (<35 mmHg)

- **Metabolic Alkalosis:**
Blood pH: >7.45
HCO3-: >26 mmHg
PaCO2: Normal or increased (>45 mmHg)

Respiratory Acidosis:

decreased lung ventilation that results in **high carbon dioxide level & low blood pH.**

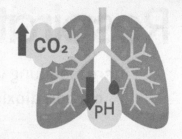

Causes:

It can occur if there is any problem with the patient's breathing rate (**too slow**), alveolar sacs (**damaged**), or diaphragm (**weak**).

Main cause: bradypnea (_depress_ed respiratory rate <12 bpm). This **causes CO2 to build up in the lungs**.

Respiratory Acidosis Lab Values:

- Blood pH: **<7.35**
- Carbon dioxide (PaCO2): **>45 mmHg**
- Bicarbonate (HCO3-): Normal or elevated (>26 mmHg)**

  - **To help compensate & correct acidosis, the kidneys can start to **conserve bicarbonate (HCO3-)** to hopefully **increase the blood's pH** back to normal.....so HCO3- can become **>26 mmHg.**

Drugs: opioids or sedatives & **d**iseases of neuromuscular system (Guillain–Barré syndrome)

Edema: pulmonary (fluid in lungs)

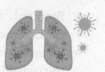

Pneumonia

Respiratory center of brain damaged (stroke)

Emphysema: overinflated alveoli

Spasms of bronchial tubes (asthma)

Sac elasticity of alveolar sac damaged (COPD)

Signs & Symptoms

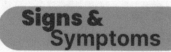

Major neurological changes:

- Confused, very drowsy, & report a headache
- Low oxygen level (**hypoxia**)
- Respiration rate **less than 12 bpm**
- **Increased** heart rate
- Hypotension
- **Increased carbon dioxide** levels

Nursing interventions

- **Administer oxygen (O2).**
  - Be careful with O2 administration in patients who have **chronic acidosis** because their body has **compensated** & is used to the high CO2 levels. A **low O2 level guides their respiratory function,** & if O2 levels go too high, their **breathing can decrease**.
- Assess **respirations** and **neuro status.**
- Encourage **coughing and deep breathing.**
- Provide **suctioning and mouth care.**
- May need respiratory treatment like **bronchodilators.**
- **Hold meds** that depress respirations (opioids etc.).
- Monitor K+ levels: respiratory acidosis can **increase potassium level** and cause **dysrhythmias.**
- Administer **antibiotics** for infection.
- May need **endotracheal intubation** if CO2 becomes severely elevated.

Respiratory Alkalosis:

increased lung ventilation that results in **low carbon dioxide level & high blood pH.**

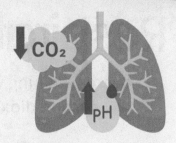

Causes:

Main cause: <u>tachypnea</u> (fast respiratory rate >20 bpm). This causes **too much CO2 to be exhaled.**

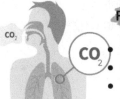

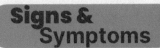

Respiratory Alkalosis Lab Values:

- Blood pH: **>7.45**
- Carbon dioxide (PaCO2): **<35 mmHg**
- Bicarbonate (HCO3-): Normal or decreased (<22 mmHg)**

To help compensate and correct alkalosis, the kidneys may start to **excrete bicarbonate (HCO3-).

The goal is to **decrease the blood's pH back to normal**.....so HCO3- can become **<22 mmHG.**

Temperature increase (**fever**)

Aspirin toxicity (**salicylates**)

Controlled ventilation excessive **(mechanical ventilation too fast)**

Hyperventilation

Yelp! (**pain, anxiety, fear**)

Pneumothorax (**collapsed lung**)

Neurological damage: inflammation of the brain or brain injury

Embolism in lungs (**clot**)

Ascending in **altitude**: low oxygen levels cause the body to hyperventilate

Signs & Symptoms

Major Sign: fast respiratory rate

- **Normal adult range:** 12-20 bpm
  - Tachypnea: >20 bpm

- **Neurological changes:** anxiety, fear, dizziness, seizures
- Increased heart rate
- Tetany, muscle cramps, dysrhythmias
  - Due to **hypocalcemia & hypokalemia**

Nursing interventions

Goal: Find cause and correct it. We want the patient to decrease breathing rate and **REST.**

Rebreather mask or paper bag to slow down breathing

Electrolytes monitored: **hypokalemia & hypocalcemia**

Sedatives or anti-anxiety meds to relieve anxiety and decrease hyperventilation

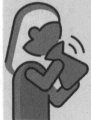

Teach relaxation and stress de-escalation techniques

Metabolic Acidosis:

increase of <u>acids</u> in the body that results in a **low blood pH and low bicarbonate level.**

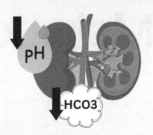

Causes:

- **Increased <u>acid</u> production**
  - **Diabetic ketoacidosis (DKA):** where **ketones** (acids) increase in the body, which decreases bicarbonate.
- **Decreased <u>acid</u> excretion**
  - **Renal failure:** there is a **high amount of waste** left in the body, which causes the acids to increase, and bicarb can't control the imbalance.
- **Loss** of too much bicarb: **diarrhea**

When this acidic phenomenon is taking place in the body, other systems will try to compensate to increase the bicarb back to normal. One system that tries to compensate is the **respiratory system**.

In order to compensate, the respiratory system will cause the body to hyperventilate by increasing breathing through **Kussmaul's respirations**.

These respirations are deep and fast. The body hopes this will help expel CO2 (an acid), which will "hopefully" increase the pH back to normal.

Accumulation of lactate leading to lactic acidosis (sepsis)

Chronic diarrhea*

Impaired renal function*

Diabetic Ketoacidosis (DKA): high ketones

Salicylates toxicity

*most common causes

Metabolic Acidosis Lab Values:

- **Blood pH:** <7.35
- **Bicarbonate (HCO3-):** <22 mmHg
- **Carbon dioxide (PaCO2):** Normal or decreased <35 mmHg, if compensating

Signs & Symptoms

Main sign: Kussmaul's respirations

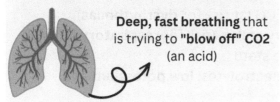

Deep, fast breathing that is trying to **"blow off"** CO2 (an acid)

- **Confused**
- **Weak**
- **Low blood pressure**
- **Cardiac changes** (hyperkalemia)

Nursing interventions

Find the cause and correct it. Interventions will vary depending on the cause:

- Monitor **respiratory system.**
- Assess other electrolyte levels:
  - Potassium: **hyperkalemia** can occur (monitor for ECG changes like tall t-waves).
  - **Hypokalemia** can occur when **acidosis resolves** due to an **extracellular to intracellular shift of K+ back into the cell**, especially with DKA.
- Diabetic ketoacidosis: IV fluids & insulin
  - monitor for **hypokalemia because insulin moves potassium inside the cell.**
- Monitor neuro status and ensure safety.
- IV fluids (vary) per doctor's order:
  - Sodium bicarbonate, 0.9% Sodium Chloride (isotonic)
- Dialysis may be needed if the patient is experiencing acidosis due to renal failure.

Metabolic Alkalosis:

decrease of acid or increase of bicarbonate in the body that results in a **high blood pH.**

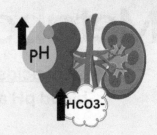

Causes:

- **Excessive loss of acids (hydrogen ions)**
- **Increased amount of bicarbonate (HCO3-)**

Metabolic Alkalosis Lab Values:

- Blood pH: **>7.45**
- Bicarbonate (HCO3-): **>26 mmHg**
- Carbon dioxide (PaCO2): Normal or increased (>45 mmHg)**

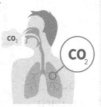

The body tries to **compensate by stimulating the **respiratory system** to **hypoventilate** (decrease respirations), which will retain PaCO2 (carbon dioxide). As a result, this will help decrease the pH back to normal, and the kidneys will start to excrete the bicarb, which will hopefully decrease the overall HCO3-.

pH scale

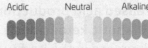

Acidic   Neutral   Alkaline

0 1 2 3 4 5 6 7 8 9 10 11 12 13 14

Acid loss via **stomach** due to suction or vomiting

Low Chloride level (increases bicarb level)

K+ loss (hypokalemia) causes wasting of CL- & increases reabsorption of HCO3-

Aldosterone elevated:
hyperaldosteronism: keep Na+, waste hydrogen ions & keep bicarb

Loop & thiazide diuretics

Infusing too much sodium bicarb IV

Signs & Symptoms

- **Bradypnea (hypoventilation)**
  - lead to respiratory failure
- **Dysrhythmias**
  - **due to hypokalemia**
- **Tetany**
- **Tremors**
- **Muscle cramping**
- **Tired**
- **Irritable**

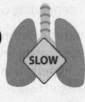

Nursing interventions

Find the cause and correct it. Interventions will vary depending on the cause:

- Monitor ECG (at risk for **dysrhythmias**), respiratory status (risk for **respiratory failure**), and neuro status.
- Monitor electrolytes: **low potassium and chloride.**
  - Administer replacement per doctor's orders.
- If vomiting, give **antiemetics** to decrease *loss of acids through emesis.*
- **Hold diuretics** that <u>worsen alkalosis</u> (loop and thiazides)
- Doctor may order **Acetazolamide (Diamox):**
  - This is a carbonic anhydrase inhibitor and a diuretic, which **reduces the reabsorption of bicarb and helps excrete it via the urine.**

Metabolic & Respiratory Acidosis/Alkalosis Test Review

1. Diabetic ketoacidosis and salicylates toxicity can lead to _____.

A. Metabolic acidosis
B. Metabolic alkalosis
C. Respiratory acidosis
D. Respiratory alkalosis

2. In metabolic alkalosis, the blood pH level is _____.

A. Decreased
B. Increased
C. Normal

3. Which of the following is NOT a cause of metabolic alkalosis?

A. Hyperaldosteronism
B. Diuretic Acetazolamide
C. Vomiting
d. Hypokalemia

4. Your patient is experiencing deep, fast respirations and has an elevated potassium level. What condition below presents with these signs and symptoms?

A. Respiratory acidosis
B. Metabolic acidosis
C. Respiratory alkalosis
D. Metabolic acidosis

5. Your patient is experiencing diabetic ketoacidosis. The doctor orders IV fluids and insulin as part of treatment. The nurse makes it a priority to monitor for what type of electrolyte imbalance?

A. Hypernatremia
B. Hyponatremia
C. Hypokalemia
D. Hyperkalemia

66

Metabolic & Respiratory Acidosis/Alkalosis Test Review

6. Which of the following is NOT a cause of respiratory acidosis?

A. Pulmonary edema
B. Asthma
C. Chronic obstructive pulmonary disease (COPD)
D. Hyperventilation

7. Your patient is post-op from knee surgery. The patient has been receiving Morphine 4 mg IV every 2 hours. You notice the patient has a respiratory rate of 8 breaths per minute and is extremely drowsy. Which condition is the patient at most risk for?

A. Respiratory acidosis
B. Respiratory alkalosis
C. Metabolic acidosis
D. Metabolic alkalosis

8. Respiratory alkalosis can affect other electrolyte levels in the body. Which of the following electrolyte levels can also be affected in this condition?

A. Calcium and sodium levels
B. Potassium and sodium levels
C. Calcium and potassium levels
D. Potassium and phosphate levels

9. Your patient is experiencing respiratory alkalosis. What is the major sign and symptom of this condition?

A. Bradypnea
B. Tachypnea
C. Bradycardia
D. Tachycardia

Metabolic & Respiratory Acidosis/Alkalosis
Answers & Rationales

1. The answer is A: metabolic acidosis. Diabetic ketoacidosis (DKA) and salicylates toxicity increase acid balance in the body, leading to metabolic acidosis.

2. The answer is B: increased. In metabolic alkalosis, the blood pH increases because either there is a decrease in acid balance in the body or an increase in bicarbonate.

3. The answer is B: Diuretic Acetazolamide. This medication is a carbonic anhydrase inhibitor, and it is a diuretic. It can be used to treat metabolic alkalosis because it reduces the reabsorption of bicarbonate, which promotes the excretion via the urine.

4. The answer is B: Metabolic acidosis. Deep, fast respirations are known as Kussmaul's respiration. This occurs as a compensatory mechanism during metabolic acidosis. It is the body's attempt to "blow off" CO2 (an acid) to help balance the blood's pH. Hyperkalemia can also present in metabolic acidosis.

5. The answer is C: Hypokalemia. Insulin administration moves potassium inside the cell and depletes blood levels. The nurse should make it a priority to monitor for low potassium levels (hypokalemia).

6. The answer is D: Hyperventilation. Hyperventilation leads to respiratory alkalosis (not acidosis) because it causes the body to expire excessive amounts of CO2. Hypoventilation (bradypnea) causes CO2 to build up in the lungs and can lead to respiratory acidosis.

7. The answer is A: Respiratory acidosis. Opioids or sedatives can lead to a depression in the respiratory rate. This can lead to the buildup of CO2 (an acid) and cause respiratory acidosis.

8. The answer is C: calcium and potassium levels.

9. The answer is B: tachypnea.

Chapter 5:
Fluid Volume Disorders

Key Terms to Know:

I'S & O'S:

- **Intake:** these are fluids taken into the body. It can be through various routes like the mouth, intravenous, or a tube.
- **Output:** These are fluids that leave the body. It can be through various routes as well, like stool, urine, emesis, and drainage.
- **Sensible loss:** aware of loss & easily measured, and includes stool, urine, emesis, GI, and wound drainage.
- **Insensible loss:** unaware of loss & hard to measure, and is the fluid that evaporates from the skin & lungs (example: water vapor you breathe out).

✎ FLUID IMBALANCES ✎

- **Fluid volume excess:** too much fluid in the body.
    - **Hypertonic overload:** increase of body water due to increase of osmolarity.
    - **Hypotonic overload:** increase of body water but not osmolarity (dilution occurs).
    - **Isotonic overload:** no movement of water from compartments because osmolarity is equal, but an increase in body water occurs in the extracellular compartment.
- **Fluid volume deficit:** not enough fluid in the body.
    - **Hypertonic dehydration:** mainly a loss of water rather than solutes (example: sodium).
    - **Hypotonic dehydration:** mainly of loss of solutes (example: sodium) rather than water.
    - **Isotonic dehydration:** equal loss of water & solutes.

Intake & Output

Water makes up **70%** of our body weight!

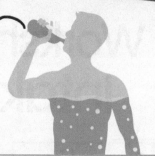

Intake

These are **FLUIDS** taken into the body. It can be through various routes like the mouth, intravenous, or a tube.

Normal Fluid <u>Intake</u> for Adults:

Liquids: 1500-2000 mL/day
Solids: 500-700 mL/day

What's Included:

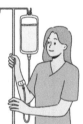

- Oral Fluids
- Intravenous Fluids & Flushes
  - Medication infusions, blood products, TPN etc.
- Tube Feedings
  - Flushes, boluses
- Irrigations
- Enemas

Oral Liquids Included:

This includes anything that is a liquid at **room temperature:**

- Juice
- Water
- Ice chips**
- Drinks (coffee, soft drinks, tea etc.)
- Milk
- Gelatin (Jell-O ®)
- Broths
- Ice cream
- Frozen treats: popsicles, sorbet
- Nutrition supplements like Ensure® or Boost ®

**Ice chips: this melts to half its volume. If you give the patient 8 mL of ice chips, record intake as 4 mL.

Output

These are **FLUIDS** that leave the body. It can be through various routes as well.

Normal Fluid <u>Output</u> for Adults:

Urine: 800-2000 mL/day
Stool: 100-250 mL/day
Insensible: 750-900 mL/day

Sensible vs. Insensible Loss:

Sensible: aware of loss & **easily measured**
  - stool, urine, emesis, GI and wound drainage
Insensible: unaware of loss & **hard to measure**
  - fluid that evaporates from skin & lungs (water vapor you breathe out)

What's Included:

- Urine
- Emesis
- Stool (liquid forms only)
  - includes ostomies
- Body drainage
  - all drains, tubes
    - example: chest tubes, wound vacs
- Suction
  - gastric and respiratory

*Insensible loss is **NOT** included in the measurement.

Worksheet 1: Calculating Intake & Output

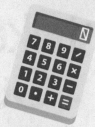

Practice

During your 7 pm-7 am shift, your patient receives the following. What is the patient's **intake** for that shift?

Time:	Fluid:
2000-0600	Jevity 50 mL/hr
0615	50 cc free water flush
2100-0215	Two 250 mL of RBCs
0115	20 cc saline flush IV
0300	Zosyn IV 50 mL
0400	10 cc saline flush IV
1900-0500	Heparin 10 mL/hr
1900-0500	Normal Saline 100 mL/hr

Intake: _____

Workspace

Answer with rationale on next page

During your 7 pm-7 am shift, your patient has the following **output**. What is the patient's output for that shift?

Ileostomy: 300 mL
NG suction: 50 cc
Urine: 1850 mL
Wound vac: 100 cc

Output: _____

Workspace

Answer with rationale on next page

71

© Nurse Sarah (RegisteredNurseRN.com)

Worksheet 1: Calculating Intake & Output Answers

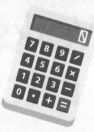

Answers

During your 7 pm-7 am shift, your patient receives the following. What is the patient's **intake** for that shift?

Time:	Fluid:
2000-0600	Jevity 50 mL/hr
0615	50 cc free water flush
2100-0215	Two 250 mL of RBCs
0115	20 cc saline flush IV
0300	Zosyn IV 50 mL
0400	10 cc saline flush IV
1900-0500	Heparin 10 mL/hr
1900-0500	Normal Saline 100 mL/hr

Intake: **2230 mL**

Workspace

2000-0600= 10 hrs
    50 ml/hr
x 10 hr
  500 mL of Jevity

250 mL
x 2
500 mL of RBCs

  10 mL/hr
x 10 hours (1900-0500)
100 mL of Heparin

  100 mL/hr
x   10 hours (1900-0500)
1000 mL of Normal Saline

500	mL	(Jevity)
50	mL	(water flush)
500	mL	(RBCs)
20	mL	(saline flush)
50	mL	(IV Zosyn)
10	mL	(saline flush)
100	mL	(Heparin)
+ 1000	mL	(NS)

2230 mL

During your 7 pm-7 am shift, your patient has the following **output**. What is the patient's output for that shift?

Ileostomy: 300 mL
NG suction: 50 cc
Urine: 1850 mL
Wound vac: 100 cc

Output: **2300 mL**

Workspace

300 mL (ileostomy)
 50 mL (NG suction)
1850 mL (urine)
+ 100 mL (wound vac)
2300 mL

Worksheet 2: Calculating Intake & Output

Practice

Calculate the patient's **intake** during your 12-hour shift:

Remember:
- 1 cc = 1 mL
- Convert oz to mL & multiply by 30

0800: Two pieces of toast, 2 cups of oatmeal, 8 oz yogurt, 12 oz orange juice, 2 oz grits

1000: Two 8 oz of coffee

1100: 24 oz of ice chips

1230: house salad, 12 oz soda

1400: One pack of red blood cells (250 mL)

1715: 10 cc saline flush IV

1600-1900: Normal Saline IV 100 cc/hr

Workspace

Intake: _____

Answer with rationale on next page

Interpreting I's and O's

Example:

Intake **4250 mL** & Output **1210 mL**
- Patient is at risk for fluid volume overload.

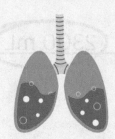

- If the intake is LESS than output or if the output is MORE than the intake, think **DEHYDRATION!**

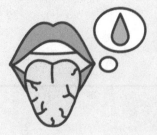

- If the intake is MORE than output or if the output is LESS than the intake, think **FLUID OVERLOAD!**

Worksheet 2: Calculating Intake & Output Answers

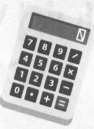

Answers

Calculate the patient's **intake** during your 12-hour shift:

0800: Two pieces of toast, 2 cups of oatmeal, 8 oz yogurt, 12 oz orange juice, 2 oz grits

1000: Two 8 oz of coffee

1100: 24 oz of ice chips

1230: house salad, 12 oz soda

1400: One pack of red blood cells (250 mL)

1715: 10 cc saline flush IV

1600-1900: Normal Saline IV 100 cc/hr

Intake: 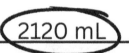 2120 mL

Workspace

12 oz
x 30 mL
360 mL (orange juice)

2 x 8 oz= 16 oz (coffee)
    x 30 mL
    480 mL (coffee)

24 oz = 12 oz (half the ice chips)
2   x 30 mL
     360 mL (ice chips)

12 oz
x 30 mL
360 mL (soda)

1600-1900 = 3 hours
100 mL
x 3 hrs.
300 mL Normal Saline

360 mL (orange juice)
480 mL (coffee)
360 mL (ice chips)
360 mL (soda)
250 mL (RBCs)
  10 mL (saline flush)
+ 300 mL (normal saline)
2120 mL

Not included:
toast, oatmeal, yogurt, grits, house salad

74

© Nurse Sarah (RegisteredNurseRN.com)

Fluid Volume Excess: too much **fluid** in the body

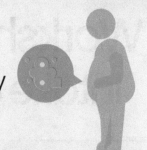

Types:

Hypertonic Overload:

- **Increase** of body water due to **increase** of osmolarity
- Leads to the movement of water from **intracellular to extracellular compartment**
- **Overloads** extracellular compartment
- **Causes:**
  - Excessive intake of **sodium**
  - **Hypertonic** IV solutions

Hypotonic Overload:
(water intoxication)

- **Increase** of body water but **NOT** osmolarity (**dilution occurs**)
- Leads to the movement of water from **extracellular to intracellular compartment**
- **Overloads** both compartments
- **Causes:**
  - Excessive intake of **free water: primary polydipsia**
  - **SIADH:** too much **ADH** being released & **water is retained**

Isotonic Overload:

- No movement of water from compartments because osmolarity is **equal**
- **Increase** in body water occurs in **extracellular compartment only**
- **Causes:**
  - **Heart** failure
  - **Kidney** failure
  - Too much **IV fluids** (isotonic)
  - **Corticosteroids:** retain sodium & water

Signs & Symptoms

- Confusion
- Headache
- Strong pulse
- ↑ heart rate
- ↑ blood pressure
- JVD
- Dyspnea
- Crackles
- ↑ respiratory rate
- Dry, hacking cough
- Edema: pitting
- Cool skin
- Ascites
- Weight gain

> **LATE:** frothy, blood-tinged

Labs & Diagnostics

Too much fluid is going to **DILUTE** everything: blood and urine diluted

> Remember **D** for **d**ilute & **d**ecreased

- **D**ecreased Hbg & Hct
- **D**ecreased sodium
- **D**ecreased BUN
- **D**ecreased urine: specific gravity & osmolality
- **D**ecreased serum osmolality (blood)

Nursing interventions
"**Drain**" the water

Diuretics: remove extra fluid via **kidneys** (loop, osmotic, thiazides)

Restrict Na+ & Fluid → **1-2 L fluid** restriction & **low sodium** foods

Assess DAILY weights (indicator of fluid status) → **1 kg=1 L of fluid** **Same** time & scale 🚫 **Gain 2-3 lbs.** in day

Intake & output **strict**

Na+ level **monitored** along w/ other electrolytes..ex: **K+**: loops can waste too much

Fluid Volume Deficit: **not enough fluid** in the body

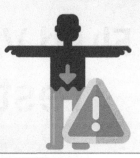

Types:

Hypertonic Dehydration:

- **Mainly** a loss of **WATER** rather than solutes (sodium)
- Also known as **hypernatremic**
- **Extracellular compartment** becomes very concentrated w/ solutes (especially sodium) and has <u>less water</u>
- **Result:** water moves from the intracellular to the extracellular compartment & the cell **SHRINKS** & become dehydrated
- Treatement: Rehydrate cell w/ hypotonic solutions
- **Causes:**
  - **Losing water:** diarrhea/vomiting, diabetes insipidus
  - **Not** taking in **enough water**

Hypotonic Dehydration:

- **Mainly** a loss of **SOLUTES** (sodium) rather than water
- Also known as **hyponatremic**
- **Extracellular compartment** has less solutes & is mainly water
- **Result:** water moves from extracellular to the intracellular compartment: cell **SWELLS** & **depletes** intravascular space
- Treatment: Add back solutes with hypertonic solutions
- **Causes:**
  - Thiazide diuretics (waste Na+)
  - IV fluids w/ **LOW solutes**: hypotonic solutions
  - Starvation/malnourished

Isotonic Dehydration:

- **EQUAL** loss of water & solutes
- **No drastic shifting** of water between compartments
- Most **common** type
- **Result:** intravascular loss that can progress to **hypovolemic shock**
- **Causes:**
  - **Diuretics**
  - **Third spacing:** water shifts from intravascular space to interstitial (can deplete intravascular)
  - **Bleeding** out (trauma)
  - Vomiting, diarrhea, sweating

Signs & Symptoms

Dry mucous membranes (no tears when crying)

Early sign: ↑heart rate (feels weak)

Hypotension (orthostatic) → **BP drops** when going from **supine** or **sitting** position to **standing position**.

Young babies: **sunken fontanelles**

Decreased skin turgor ****not a sign for geriatric pts.**

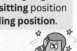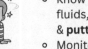

Refill to capillaries sluggish (>3 sec.)
**not a sign for geriatric pts.

Attitude changes (restless, confused, lethargic)

Thirsty ****not a sign for geriatric & young children pts.**

Experience **weight loss**

Diagnostics (labs)

↑ serum osmolality
↑ hbg & hct
↑ BUN
↑ Na+ level
↑ urine osmolality
↑ Urine specific gravity

*lab results depend on type of dehydration

Nursing interventions

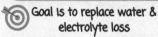 Goal is to replace water & electrolyte loss

- Weigh patient **DAILY**
  - same time, same scale
  - gaining weight or losing?
  - great **early indicator** of patient's fluid status
- **Strict** intake and output tracking:
  - Know exactly what patient is **taking in** (IV fluids, flushes, oral & tube feedings, irrigation) & **putting out** (urine, vomit, suction etc.).
  - Monitor **urinary output closely** to make sure hydration status is improving: **30 mL/hr or 0.5 mL/kg/hr**
- Treat w/ **oral hydration** & administering **IV fluids** per doctor's order:
  - Type of IV fluids used **depends on the cause.**
  - *Typically* isotonic fluids, **but** if hypertonic dehydration, hypotonic fluids may be used. If hypotonic dehydration, hypertonic fluids may be used.
- Monitor electrolyte levels (sodium).

Fluid Volume Overload & Excess Test Review

1. The patient is experiencing a severe case of SIADH (Syndrome of Inappropriate Antidiuretic Hormone). What type of overload is the patient most likely to experience?

A. Hypertonic overload
B. Hypotonic overload
C. Isotonic overload

2. What type of fluid volume overload occurs because water moves from the intracellular to the extracellular compartment due to an increase in osmolarity of extracellular fluid, which increases body water?

A. Hypertonic overload
B. Hypotonic overload
C. Isotonic overload

3. A patient is experiencing hypertonic overload. What could cause this type of overload?

A. Corticosteroids over usage
B. Primary polydipsia
C. SIADH
D. Excessive sodium intake

4. What type of fluid volume overload presents with no drastic shifting of water from the compartments because osmolarity is equal but overloads the extracellular compartment?

A. Hypertonic overload
B. Hypotonic overload
C. Isotonic overload

77

Fluid Volume Overload & Excess Test Review

5. Select all the signs and symptoms below that could present with fluid overload:

A. Weight gain
B. >3 seconds capillary refill
C. Orthostatic hypotension
D. Frothy, bloody tinged cough
E. Ascites
F. Jugular venous distention
G. Weak pulse
H. Rales

6. Your patient has a diagnosis of fluid volume overload (isotonic). Select all the interventions you plan to implement for this patient:

A. Encourage patient to limit fluid intake to 4 liters per day
B. Strict monitoring of intake and output
C. Weigh patient daily at the same time with the same scale
D. Administer diuretics per physician's order
E. Ensure urinary output is at least 10 mL/hr or greater
F. Restrict foods high in sodium

7. Your patient, who is receiving treatment for fluid volume overload, has lost 2 lbs. since receiving treatment. Based on the patient's weight loss, about how much fluid has the patient lost?

A. 2 liters
B. 6 liters
C. 4 liters
D. 1 liter

Fluid Volume Overload & Excess Test Review

8. You assess the lab report for your patient who has isotonic fluid volume overload. Which lab results below are expected with this condition? Select all that apply:

A. Decreased hemoglobin
B. Increased sodium level
C. Decreased urine specific gravity
D. Increased BUN
E. Decreased serum osmolality

9. What type of dehydration presents with mainly a loss of water rather than electrolytes (solutes)?

A. Hypertonic dehydration
B. Hypotonic dehydration
C. Isotonic dehydration

10. A patient with diabetes insipidus is most likely to experience what type of fluid volume deficit (dehydration)?

A. Hypertonic dehydration
B. Hypotonic dehydration
C. Isotonic dehydration

11. What type of dehydration presents mainly with a loss of electrolytes (solutes) rather than water?

A. Hypertonic dehydration
B. Hypotonic dehydration
C. Isotonic dehydration

Fluid Volume Overload & Excess Test Review

12. Your patient is experiencing a severe gastrointestinal bleed. What type of fluid volume deficit will this patient experience?

A. Hypertonic dehydration
B. Hypotonic dehydration
C. Isotonic dehydration

13. What signs and symptoms of fluid volume deficit are not a reliable indicator in older adults (geriatric patient populations)? Select all that apply:

A. Hypotension
B. Confusion
C. Thirst
D. Weight loss
E. Decreased skin turgor

14. What signs and symptoms in a young infant would alert the nurse that the patient is likely experiencing fluid volume deficit? Select all that apply:

A. Weight gain
B. Bulging fontanelles
C. Sunken fontanelles
D. No tears when crying

15. A patient is admitted with fluid volume deficit (isotonic dehydration). What lab results would the nurse expect to see in this patient? Select all that apply:

A. Decreased hemoglobin
B. Increased serum osmolality
C. Increased urine specific gravity
D. Decreased urine osmolality
E. Increased BUN

Fluid Volume Overload & Excess Test Review

16. A patient is receiving treatment for fluid volume deficit (hypertonic dehydration). What will the nurse implement in the patient's plan of care? Select all that apply:

A. Daily weights
B. Administer hypotonic IV solutions per physician's order
C. Increase sodium intake
D. Monitor sodium level
E. Encourage the patient to limit fluids to 1-2 liters per day
F. Strict intake and output measurements

17. What signs and symptoms could present with fluid volume deficit in an adult patient? Select all that apply:

A. Weight loss
B. Pitting edema
C. Confusion
D. Rales
E. Thirst
F. Orthostatic hypotension
G. Weak pulse
H. Normal skin turgor

 Answers for the questions are on the next page.

Fluid Volume Overload & Excess Answers & Rationales

1. The answer is B: hypotonic overload. In SIADH, there is too much ADH being released, and water is retained. This will increase body water and dilute the extracellular fluid (hence lowering its osmolarity). This will cause water to move from the extracellular to the intracellular compartment and overload both compartments.

2. The answer is A: hypertonic overload. Hypertonic overload occurs because water has moved from the intracellular to the extracellular compartment. This is due to an increase in osmolarity of the extracellular fluid.

3. The answer is D: excessive sodium intake. This will cause an increase of sodium concentration in the blood (plasma), which will increase osmolarity and cause hypertonic overload.

4. The answer is C. Isotonic overload presents with no drastic shifting of water from the compartments because osmolarity is equal but overloads the extracellular compartment. This can happen from heart or kidney failure, too much isotonic IV fluids, and over usage of corticosteroids (which cause the body to retain sodium and water).

5. The answers are A, D, E, F, and H. All of these are possible signs and symptoms of fluid volume overload. Option B, C, and G are signs found in fluid volume deficit.

6. The answers are B, C, D, and F. Option A is not correct because 4 L/day is a high amount of fluid, and the patient should be on a fluid restriction of about 1-2 L/day. Option E is not correct because the nurse should ensure the urinary output is at least 30 mL/hr (0.5mL/kg/day). A urinary output of >10 mL/hr is too low and not an appropriate goal for the patient.

7. The answer is D: 1 liter. A general rule to remember is that 1 kg (2.2 lbs) is equal to about 1 liter of fluid. Therefore, if the patient has lost 2 lbs., the patient has lost around 1 liter of fluid.

8. The answers are A, C, and E. Remember, when fluid volume overload is presenting, there is going to be a lot of fluid in the blood and urine. This will make the blood and

urine less concentrated (diluted). Therefore, the concentration of certain substances in the blood will be decreased. The patient can have: decrease in hemoglobin and hematocrit, decrease in sodium, decreased urine specific gravity and osmolality, and decreased serum osmolality.

9. The answer is A: hypertonic dehydration. This presents with mainly a loss of water rather than electrolytes (solutes). This is also known as hypernatremia.

10. The answer is A: hypertonic dehydration. Diabetes insipidus (DI) causes the patient to void a high volume of urine. This is due to a low level of ADH being produced in the body. DI will cause the extracellular compartment to lose mainly water rather than electrolytes. This change in osmolarity will further cause fluid to move from intracellular to extracellular compartment and shrink the cell.

11. The answer is B: hypotonic dehydration. Hypotonic dehydration presents mainly with a loss of electrolytes (solutes) rather than water. This is also known as hyponatremia.

12. The answer is C: isotonic dehydration. This type of fluid volume deficit occurs when there is an EQUAL loss of water and electrolytes. This is the most common type of fluid volume deficit seen, and the problem from this type of dehydration arises from the intravascular loss (which can lead to hypovolemic shock).

13. The answers are C and E. Thirst and decreased skin turgor are not reliable indicators of fluid volume deficit in older adults. As people age, the thirst response decreases along with skin elasticity. In addition, capillary refill can also be naturally sluggish in geriatric populations.

14. The answers are C and D. Sunken fontanelles (the spaces in between the skull bones that present as soft spots on the head during the first part of life) and no tears when crying would alert the nurse the infant is dehydrated. In addition, the infant may be fussy, restless, and experience weight loss.

Fluid Volume Overload & Excess Answers & Rationales ✓

15. The answers are B, C, and E. Lab results are going to depend on the type of dehydration, but in most cases there will be a low amount of fluid in the blood and urine. Therefore, the blood and urine are going to be concentrated. As a result, the tests that check for blood and urine concentrations will be INCREASED: serum osmolality, hemoglobin, hematocrit, BUN, sodium level, urine specific gravity, and osmolality.

16. The answers are A, B, D, and F. The nurse would want to weigh the patient daily (this is a great early indicator of the patient's fluid status); administer hypotonic IV solutions per physician's order to help rehydrate the cell and fluid compartments; and monitor sodium level because it can become too high in this type of dehydration.

However, when the nurse administers hypotonic IV solutions, the sodium level should be monitored to ensure it doesn't get too low (hyponatremia) because the hypotonic solution could dilute the fluid quickly if not monitored closely. Limiting fluids should be avoided (1-2 L/day is a low amount of fluid per day and would be initiated in fluid volume OVERLOAD). Finally, the nurse would strictly monitor intake and output to ensure the patient is receiving enough fluid and urinary output is within normal range (30 mL/hr or 0.5 mL/kg/hr).

17. The answers are A, C, E, F, and G. Weight loss, confusion, thirst, orthostatic hypotension, and weak pulse can all present in adults with fluid volume deficit. Skin turgor would be decreased (slow to bounce back), not normal.

Photo Credits & References:

Juxtaglomerular apparatus: extender_01/shutterstock.com

Blood Tests | National Heart, Lung, and Blood Institute (NHLBI). (2019). Retrieved from https://www.nhlbi.nih.gov/health-topics/blood-tests

Bradley, J. G., & Davis, K. A. (2003, December 15). Orthostatic hypotension. American Family Physician. Retrieved April 28, 2023, from https://www.aafp.org/pubs/afp/issues/2003/1215/p2393.html

Burger MK, Schaller DJ. Metabolic Acidosis. [Updated 2022 Jul 19]. In: StatPearls [Internet]. Treasure Island (FL): StatPearls Publishing; 2023 Jan-. Available from: https://www.ncbi.nlm.nih.gov/books/NBK482146/

Carter, P. (2007). Lippincott's Textbook for Nursing Assistants (2nd ed., p. 403). Lippincott Williams & Wilkins.

Center for Food Safety and Applied Nutrition. (2022, February 25). Sodium in your diet. U.S. Food and Drug Administration. https://www.fda.gov/food/nutrition-education-resources-materials/sodium-your-diet

Centers for Disease Control and Prevention. (2022, August 23). Sodium, Potassium and Health. Centers for Disease Control and Prevention. https://www.cdc.gov/salt/potassium.htm

Chen I, Lui F. Physiology, Active Transport. [Updated 2022 Sep 12]. In: StatPearls [Internet]. Treasure Island (FL): StatPearls Publishing; 2023 Jan-. Available from: https://www.ncbi.nlm.nih.gov/books/NBK547718/

Chloride in diet: MedlinePlus Medical Encyclopedia. Medlineplus.gov. (2021). Retrieved 29 November 2021, from https://medlineplus.gov/ency/article/002417.htm.

Comprehensive Metabolic Panel (CMP): MedlinePlus Lab Test Information. (2020). Retrieved 21 April 2020, from https://medlineplus.gov/lab-tests/comprehensive-metabolic-panel-cmp/

Cooper GM. The Cell: A Molecular Approach. 2nd edition. Sunderland (MA): Sinauer Associates; 2000. Transport of Small Molecules. Available from: https://www.ncbi.nlm.nih.gov/books/NBK9847/

Dengue Clinical Case Management E-learning. (2023). Crystalloid & Colloid IV Solutions: Intravenous Fluids. Retrieved from https://www.cdc.gov/dengue/training/cme/ccm/page70749.html.

Fountain JH, Lappin SL. Physiology, Renin Angiotensin System. [Updated 2019 May 5]. In: StatPearls [Internet]. Treasure Island (FL): StatPearls Publishing; 2019 Jan-. Available from: https://www.ncbi.nlm.nih.gov/books/NBK470410

Hopkins E, Sanvictores T, Sharma S. Physiology, Acid Base Balance. [Updated 2022 Sep 12]. In: StatPearls [Internet]. Treasure Island (FL): StatPearls Publishing; 2023 Jan-. Available from: https://www.ncbi.nlm.nih.gov/books/NBK507807/

Photo Credits & References:

Hydrostatic pressure: Meaning and examples of use. Hydrostatic Pressure | meaning and examples of use. (n.d.). https://dictionary.cambridge.org/us/example/english/hydrostatic-pressure

Insensible water loss. (2018) Mosby's Medical Dictionary, 8th edition. (2009). Retrieved February 8 2018 from https://medical-dictionary.thefreedictionary.com/insensible+water+loss

Leib DE, Zimmerman CA, Knight ZA. Thirst. Curr Biol. 2016 Dec 19;26(24):R1260-R1265. doi: 10.1016/j.cub.2016.11.019. PMID: 27997832; PMCID: PMC5957508.

Lopez MJ, Hall CA. Physiology, Osmosis. [Updated 2023 Mar 13]. In: StatPearls [Internet]. Treasure Island (FL): StatPearls Publishing; 2023 Jan-. Available from: https://www.ncbi.nlm.nih.gov/books/NBK557609/

Merriam-Webster. (n.d.). Osmolarity. In Merriam-Webster.com dictionary. Retrieved March 08, 2023, from https://www.merriam-webster.com/dictionary/osmolarity

National Institutes of Health. (2001). National Cholesterol Education Program: ATP III Guidelines At-A-Glance Quick Desk Reference [Ebook] (pp. 1-2).

NCI Dictionary: Aldosterone. National Cancer Institute. (n.d.). https://www.cancer.gov/publications/dictionaries/cancer-terms/def/aldosterone

Shrimanker I, Bhattarai S. Electrolytes. [Updated 2021 Jul 26]. In: StatPearls [Internet]. Treasure Island (FL): StatPearls Publishing; 2021 Jan-. Available from: https://www.ncbi.nlm.nih.gov/books/NBK541123/

Taylor K, Jones EB. Adult Dehydration. [Updated 2022 Oct 3]. In: StatPearls [Internet]. Treasure Island (FL): StatPearls Publishing; 2023 Jan-. Available from: https://www.ncbi.nlm.nih.gov/books/NBK555956/

The A1C Test & Diabetes | NIDDK. Retrieved from https://www.niddk.nih.gov/health-information/diabetes/overview/tests-diagnosis/a1c-test

The capillary wall (2018, July) Centers for Disease Control and Prevention. Available at: https://www.cdc.gov/dengue/training/cme/ccm/page71620.html.

U.S. Department of Health and Human Services. NIH: Understand Your Complete Blood Count (CBC) and Common Blood Deficiencies [Ebook] (p. 1). Bethesda.

U.S. National Library of Medicine. (2021, November 6). Fluid imbalance: Medlineplus medical encyclopedia. MedlinePlus. https://medlineplus.gov/ency/article/001187.htm

Weir MR, Dzau VJ. The renin-angiotensin-aldosterone system: a specific target for hypertension management. Am J Hypertens. 1999 Dec;12(12 Pt 3):205S-213S. doi: 10.1016/s0895-7061(99)00103-x. PMID: 10619573.

III, J. L. L. (2023, April 18). Volume overload - endocrine and metabolic disorders. Merck Manuals Professional Edition. https://www.merckmanuals.com/professional/endocrine-and-metabolic-disorders/fluid-metabolism/volume-overload

Made in the USA
Coppell, TX
04 October 2023